12

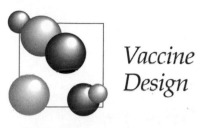

Vaccine
Design

Molecular Medical Science Series

Series Editors

Keith James, University of Edinburgh Medical School, UK
Alan Morris, University of Warwick, UK

Forthcoming Titles in the Series

Molecular Genetics of Human Inherited Disease *edited by* D.J. Shaw
Molecular Aspects of Bacterial Virulence *edited by* S. Patrick and M. Larkin
Molecular Techniques in Histopathology *edited by* J. Crocker

OtherTitles in the Series

Plasma and Recombinant Blood Products in Medical Therapy *edited by* C.V. Prowse
Introduction to the Molecular Genetics of Cancer *edited by* R.G. Vile
The Molecular Biology of Immunosuppression *edited by* A.W. Thomson
Molecular Aspects of Dermatology *edited by* G.C. Priestley
Molecular and Antibody Probes in Diagnosis *edited by* M.R Walker and R. Rapley

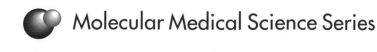 Molecular Medical Science Series

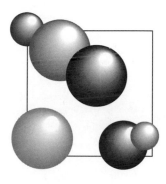

Vaccine Design

F. BROWN
Yale University, USA

G. DOUGAN
Director, Centre for Biotechnology, Imperial College,
University of London, UK

E. M. HOEY
Lecturer, School of Biology and Biochemistry,
Queen's University of Belfast, UK

S. J. MARTIN
Director, School of Biology and Biochemistry,
Queen's University of Belfast, UK

B. K. RIMA
Reader, School of Biology and Biochemistry,
Queen's University of Belfast, UK

A. TRUDGETT
Senior Research Officer, School of Biology and Biochemistry,
Queen's University of Belfast, UK

JOHN WILEY & SONS
Chichester · New York · Brisbane · Toronto · Singapore

Published 1993 by John Wiley & Sons Ltd,
            Baffins Lane, Chichester,
            West Sussex PO19 1UD, England

Other Wiley Editorial Offices

John Wiley & Sons, Inc., 605 Third Avenue,
New York, NY 10158-0012, USA

Jacaranda Wiley Ltd, G.P.O. Box 859, Brisbane,
Queensland 4001, Australia

John Wiley & Sons (Canada) Ltd, 22 Worcester Road,
Rexdale, Ontario M9W 1L1, Canada

John Wiley & Sons (SEA) Pte Ltd, 37 Jalan Pemimpin #05-04,
Block B, Union Industrial Building, Singapore 2057

Library of Congress Cataloging-in-Publication Data

Vaccine design / F. Brown ... [et al.].
      p.   cm.—(Molecular medical science series)
      Includes bibliographical references and index.
      ISBN 0 471 93727 4
      1. Synthetic vaccines.   2. Vaccines—Design.   I. Brown, Fred,
1925-   . II. Series.
      [DNLM: 1. Vaccines.   2. Drug Design.   QW 805 V1158 1993]
      QR189.2..V3   1993
      615' .372—dc20
      DNLM/DLC
      for Library of Congress   93-9132
                                                                    CIP

British Library Cataloguing in Publication Data

A catalogue record for this book is available from the British Library

ISBN 0 471 93727 4

Typeset in 10/12pt Palatino from authors' disks by Text Processing Department,
John Wiley & Sons Ltd, Chichester
Printed and bound in Great Britain by Biddles Ltd, Guildford, Surrey

Contents

1 A Short History of Vaccination

In this chapter we will look at the history of vaccination and trace its roots from early practices in India and China until the definitive and critical experiments of Jenner in 1798, which have been the basis of vaccinology for the past 200 years.

THE ORIGINS OF VACCINATION

Edward Jenner, a country doctor living in Berkeley in the south-west of England at the turn of the eighteenth century, is given the credit for 'inventing' vaccination. Although this claim has considerable justification, very few inventions can be attributed to one person and this is certainly true of vaccination. What is equally true, however, is that invention depends on the power of observation, and Jenner possessed this in no small measure. Stimulated and inspired by John Hunter, with whom he had served his apprenticeship at St George's Hospital in London, Jenner made several notable observations. One of these was the parasitic behaviour of the young cuckoo and, in fact, it was for this observation that he was elected to the Fellowship of the Royal Society in 1789.

In the context of this book, however, his massive contribution towards the control of smallpox concerns us most. The first descriptions of the control of smallpox are attributed to the Indians in the tenth century (Henderson, 1988). The disease was devastating and of those who contracted it about 25% died. The Indians observed that considerable control of the disease could be obtained by deliberately inoculating or insoufflating patients with extracts from scabs taken from people who had recovered from the illness. Although this practice still resulted in a mortality rate of about 1%, its use spread to China and other countries in that part of the world. The practice, which was known as variolation, continued for many centuries but knowledge of it only seems to have reached the Western world at the beginning of the eighteenth century. A letter to a Dr Martin Lister (a Fellow of the Royal Society) from an East India Company trader stationed in China and a report to the Royal Society of the Chinese practice by Dr Clopton Havers in 1700 seem to be the first records of the practice to have reached Europe. Several years later, on 27th May 1714, Dr John Woodward reported to the Society extracts of a letter from a Dr Emanuele Timoni, the family physician to the British Ambassador to Turkey, describing inoculation as a familiar practice among the Turks. This report aroused sufficient interest for the Society to seek further information from the British Consul to Smyrna, which resulted in the publication 2 years later of a more extensive description of the practice prepared in 1716 by Dr Jacobo Pylarini, then serving as Venetian Consul in Smyrna. Pylarini confirmed the efficacy and relative safety of the practice. It seems, however, that Lady Mary Wortley Montagu, the wife of the British Ambassador to Turkey, was probably more influential and energetic in drawing attention to its value. There is the famous letter to Sarah Chiswell in 1717 which included the following sentence: 'The smallpox so fatal and so general among us, is here entirely harmless by the invention of ingrafting which is the term they give it.' On her return to England in 1719 she clearly influenced the Prince and Princess of Wales in reaching the decision to have two of their daughters vaccinated—but not of course before the method had been tried out on six condemned criminals in Newgate prison.

Both 'experiments' were successful, and the publicity they engendered led to the temporary popularity of the procedure. However, there was considerable opposition and variolation did not 'catch on'. Doubtless the fact that the practice itself claimed many victims led to this reluctance, but it cannot be emphasised too strongly that smallpox claimed thousands of lives each year in many countries at that time. Consequently any action which led to a reduction in the number of victims was to be applauded.

In the early days the practice tended to be confined to the upper classes. Nevertheless, the principle which had been established many centuries before, that considerable success could be achieved by variolation, was confirmed. However, it was the observation that milkmaids rarely contracted smallpox that heralded the start of vaccination as we understand it today. This immunity was attributed to the fact that milkmaids contracted cowpox during milking, usually causing lesions on their hands, which protected them against the disease. Consequently milkmaids had a fair skin lacking the pock marks left on those who contracted smallpox but then recovered from the disease.

> 'Where are you going my pretty maid?'
> 'I'm going a-milking, Sir,' she said.

There are several records in the second half of the eighteenth century which point to the value of using cowpox to prevent smallpox. Probably the best documented is that of Benjamin Jesty, a farmer of Downshay in Wiltshire who inoculated his wife Elizabeth and two of their three young children with cowpox in 1774. However, it was Jenner, two decades later, who first carried out critical experiments which showed that inoculation with cowpox protected the recipients against challenge or subsequent infection with smallpox. But the number of recipients he tested in this way was small and the Royal Society rejected his paper on the subject.

Consequently the first description of the practice was published privately by Jenner in his famous Inquiry (Jenner, 1798).

THE GOLDEN AGE OF MICROBIOLOGY

It was not until almost a century later that immunisation against other infectious diseases began. Then, in rapid succession between 1880 and 1885, Pasteur demonstrated the efficacy of the vaccines he and his colleagues prepared against chicken cholera, anthrax and rabies. The publicity surrounding the demonstration of the value of the anthrax vaccine at Pouilly-le-Fort near Paris and the post-exposure protection of Joseph Meister and Jean Baptiste Jupille, both of whom had been severely bitten by a rabid dog in France, ignited the interest of those responsible for public health. At the same time, there was a rapid growth in our knowledge of the causal agents of many infectious agents, led by the founders of microbiology, Koch in Germany and Pasteur in France. The agents causing anthrax, diphtheria, tetanus, tuberculosis and the plague were isolated in rapid succession and efforts were made to produce vaccines against them.

Of particular significance was the demonstration that it was not necessary for the causal agent to multiply in the host in order to achieve protection. Although there was confusion in the identification of the organism causing hog cholera, around 1886 it was demonstrated that heat-inactivated cultures of *Salmonella choleraesuis* would protect experimental animals against infection, and by the turn of the century killed vaccines had been prepared against cholera, plague and typhoid. These were used on a limited scale, generally in order to control an outbreak of the disease. However, after a trial in more than 2000 personnel in the Indian Army, Almroth Wright was allowed to use the typhoid fever vaccine he had prepared prophylactically to immunise troops embarking for the Boer War in South Africa, despite the adverse side reactions it was known to produce.

But probably of greater importance, as we move towards vaccines based on subunits of microorganisms, was the demonstration that the secreted toxins of the organisms causing diphtheria and tetanus elicited antibody which, when passively transferred, protected patients suffering from these diseases. The classical work of Behring and Kitasato with diphtheria antitoxin led to the first Nobel Prize for Physiology or Medicine in 1901. Twenty-five years later Ramon and Glenny and their colleagues showed that active immunisation against these diseases could be achieved by inoculation of the detoxified toxins. These products were the first subunit vaccines although this description is rarely, if ever, used in describing them.

The golden age of discovery in microbiology continued into the early years of the twentieth century with the identification of the causal agents of many human and animal diseases. A major step was the recognition that filterable agents would cause disease. The pioneering work was done with tobacco mosaic virus by Ivanovski in 1892 and Beijerinck in 1897 and from these studies emerged the important fact that viruses were not simply small bacteria but differed from them in several important properties, the principal one of which is that viruses are essentially molecules requiring the full apparatus of the cell for their replication. The first disease of animals, that was shown by Loeffler and Frosch in 1898 to be caused by a virus was foot-and-mouth disease. Following this demonstration, the agents causing such important diseases as poliomyelitis, measles, smallpox and yellow fever were soon identified as viruses.

THE MODERN ERA

Experimental vaccines against many of these virus diseases were prepared. These experiments demonstrated that protection could be induced by using either weakened strains of the agents or the virulent agents that had been suitably inactivated. What was lacking was the means to grow them in the large amounts required for vaccine production. Nevertheless, Theiler and Smith in 1937 successfully produced a vaccine in hen eggs against yellow fever which was not only highly effective but was also very safe.

The impetus for producing virus vaccines on the scale required for large-scale vaccination came from the discovery of antibiotics. Although the culture of viruses outside the animal body had been demonstrated in the early 1930s in small-scale experiments, the expansion of these methods in large-scale culture proved impossible until the advent of antibiotics. It is Frenkel, a major figure in the development of foot-and-mouth disease vaccines, to whom credit should be given because of his demonstration that a virus could be produced in sufficient quantities outside the animal body for use as a vaccine. Frenkel in 1947 produced foot-and-mouth disease virus in fragments of surviving bovine tongue epithelium in quantities sufficient for it to be used, after inactivation with formaldehyde, for the first comprehensive vaccination programme initiated in Holland in 1952. This development was soon adopted by other countries in Western Europe, and its success can be judged by the knowledge that no outbreak has occurred in Western Europe since 1989. Whether it is wise for the European Community to have stopped vaccination against the disease from the beginning of 1992 remains to be seen.

The development of large-scale tissue culture techniques led to the production of many more viral vaccines; that against poliomyelitis was particularly noteworthy because it was the first human vaccine in the post-Second World War era. Since that highly dramatic time in the mid-1950s several new vaccines have been introduced, and the incidence of measles, mumps, rubella and of course poliomyelitis has been greatly reduced in the industrialised countries. There are equally successful experiences in veterinary medicine, with highly effective vaccines against rabies, rinderpest, Newcastle disease and Marek's disease, in addition to the foot-and-mouth vaccine already mentioned.

While there is no doubting the value of vaccination in preventing many of the dangerous infectious diseases of man and his domesticated and pet animals, there are still some problems in the use of the products which are currently available, as is summarised in Tables 1.1 and 1.2.

Table 1.1 Disadvantages with live-attenuated vaccines

1. Possible presence of adventitious agents in the cells and medium used for growth
2. Reversion to virulence which causes a small but significant number of clinical cases each year
3. Refrigerator temperatures are required for storage and transport
4. Limited shelf-life

Table 1.2 Disadvantages with killed vaccines

1. Hazard to personnel working with large amounts of human pathogens (e.g. rabies virus)
2. Hazard to the environment when working with large amounts of virus which will infect livestock (e.g. foot-and-mouth disease virus)
3. Need to ensure complete inactivation of infectivity
4. Presence of considerable amounts of cellular material, leading to side-effects (e.g. the rabies vaccine produced in the brains of sheep and goats can cause neurological problems in man; foot-and-mouth disease vaccine produced in tissue culture cells can cause hypersensitivity and anaphylaxis in cattle)
5. More than one injection usually required
6. Refrigerator temperatures are required for storage and transport
7. Limited shelf-life

THE IMPACT OF RECOMBINANT DNA TECHNOLOGIES

Moreover, there are diseases such as malaria and hepatitis for which conventional attenuated and inactivated vaccines are not available because the causal agents cannot be grown in sufficient amounts to allow the classical methods to be used. In addition the hazard to personnel and the immediate environment when large amounts of virulent organisms such as that causing rabies are being handled is abundantly clear. Confronted with these problems, recombinant DNA techniques are starting to play a direct role in the development of new vaccines. As mentioned above, it has been known for almost a century that the complete organism is not required to achieve protection against diphtheria or tetanus. Arguably the toxins secreted by these bacteria were our first subunit vaccines. As the molecular approach began to make an impact on virology it was demonstrated in the 1960s that protective immune responses could be elicited by individual proteins obtained from virus particles by gentle disruption. These observations, together with the parallel increase in information on the genomic organisation of many viruses, and consequently the identification of the genes coding for the immunogenic proteins, are enabling vaccination procedures to be studied in a more rational and detailed way. Added to this is the staggering increase in our knowledge of the immune response at the molecular and structural levels.

SUMMARY

We are thus at a very interesting point in the history of the development of vaccines. Although with the exception of a vaccine for hepatitis B the practical benefits of these studies have yet to be realised, it now appears likely that spectacular advances will be made in the near future. Young scientists willing to cross the traditional boundaries of microbiology, genetics, biochemistry, immunology, chemistry and physics, and attempt to understand more about the immune response and the subtle influence of shape and form of antigens and epitopes, will find an exciting future in opening up new horizons for both therapy and prophylaxis in medical and veterinary fields in the next century.

SUGGESTED READING

Henderson DA (1988) Smallpox and vaccinia. In: Plotkin SA and Mortimer EA (eds) *Vaccines*, Ch. 2, pp. 8–30. Philadelphia: Saunders.
Jenner E (1798) An inquiry into the causes and effects of the variolae vaccinae, a disease discovered in some of the western counties of England, particularly Gloucestershire and known by the name of smallpox. London: Samson Low.

2 Sequence Analysis: A Starting Point for Vaccine Design

INTRODUCTION

In order to understand the antigenic structure of any particular pathogen at the molecular level it is necessary to know the primary sequence of the proteins which contribute to it. Since it is difficult and costly to sequence proteins directly the development of nucleic acid cloning and sequencing techniques have been crucial in this respect. For example, the genes for the structural proteins of various viruses have been sequenced and the inferred amino acid sequences obtained. In some instances sequence comparisons between closely related but antigenically distinct strains have indicated variable regions which may be possible *antigenic sites*. In other cases antigenic sites have been identified by sequencing the genomes of escape mutants obtained by growing the virus in the presence of neutralising *monoclonal antibodies*. In addition, knowledge of the genome sequence is necessary for the design and construction of recombinant chimeric viruses which may have potential use as vaccines. Thus cloning and sequencing techniques have become not only powerful tools for increasing our knowledge of the antigenic structure of various infectious agents but are basic requirements for the development of novel methods of vaccine design.

Figure 2.1 shows the various steps involved in the design of a modern vaccine. Steps 1 and 2 are described in Chapters 3 and 4. Step 6 is discussed in Chapter 5 and step 7 in Chapter 4. Various means of expressing proteins (step 8) and the production of chimeric viruses (step 9) are mentioned in Chapter 9. The current chapter will consider briefly the basic cloning strategies and the principal methods for determining nucleic acid and amino acid sequences and deals mainly with steps 3, 4 and 5. Readers who are already familiar with cloning and sequencing procedures may wish to continue with Chapter 3.

NUCLEIC ACID CLONING TECHNIQUES

The starting material for cloning experiments can be either RNA or DNA; however, different strategies have to be employed depending on which nucleic acid is used. These will be dealt with in turn.

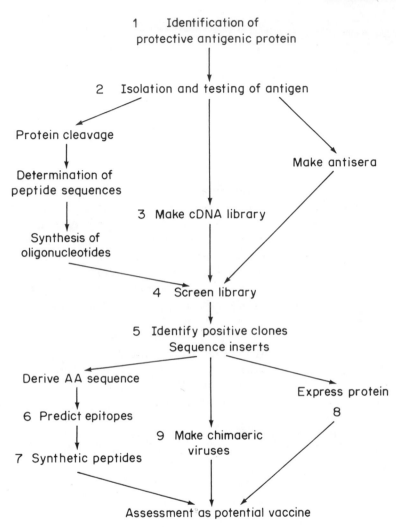

1   Identification of
protective antigenic protein

2   Isolation and testing of antigen

Protein cleavage

Determination of
peptide sequences

Make antisera

3   Make cDNA library

Synthesis of
oligonucleotides

4   Screen library

5   Identify positive clones
Sequence inserts

Derive AA sequence

Express protein
8

6   Predict epitopes

9   Make chimaeric
viruses

7   Synthetic peptides

Assessment as potential vaccine

Fig. 2.1 The main steps involved in novel vaccine design. The numbers refer to procedures which are described in various chapters of this book

CLONING FROM RNA

RNA cannot be cloned directly; therefore it is necessary first to make a complementary DNA (cDNA) copy. The enzyme that is used for this is reverse transcriptase, an RNA-dependent DNA polymerase. A primer which anneals to the RNA to be transcribed is required and synthesis is initiated from the 3′ end. The primer can be oligo dT if 3′-polyadenylated mRNA species are being reverse transcribed, or alternatively it may be possible to generate a primer specific for a particular species of RNA if part of the sequence is already known. Where neither is the case, short random nucleotide sequences may be used. Following reverse transcription double-stranded RNA/cDNA molecules are generated. Usually the RNA strand is then removed and the cDNA is made double-stranded prior to cloning. A variety of methods can be used for this but only one, which possibly has become the most popular—the Gubler and Hoffman method—is described

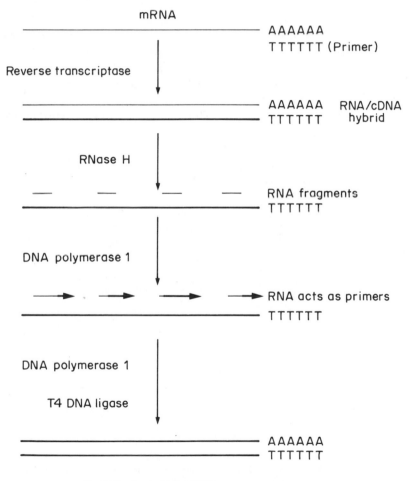

Fig. 2.2 Synthesis of double-stranded DNA from mRNA. Following synthesis of first strand cDNA using reverse transcriptase, gaps are introduced into the RNA template by RNase H. The remaining primers act as primers for DNA polymerase 1 and the gaps are sealed using a DNA ligase

here (Fig. 2.2). A combination of three enzymes is used. The first, RNase H, specifically hydrolyses RNA in the RNA/cDNA hybrid, introducing gaps. The remaining short RNA fragments, still annealed to the template, act as primers for a DNA polymerase enzyme which fills in the gaps. Finally a DNA ligase enzyme is used to seal the gaps covalently. To ensure that the resulting DNA is blunt-ended, a further treatment is often carried out with T4 DNA polymerase to remove any remaining single-stranded ends.

The double-stranded cDNA generated by the method described above can be cloned directly following ligation to a vector opened at a suitable restriction site. However, the efficiency of ligation and thus of cloning is low; consequently alternative methods have been developed to overcome this. One method used extensively in the past is to create homopolymeric tails (13–15 nucleotides in length) on the 3' ends of the DNA using the enzyme terminal deoxynucleotidyl transferase in the presence of a single deoxynucleotide triphosphate. The vector for insertion (generally a plasmid) is cleaved with the appropriate restriction enzyme and a complementary homopolymeric tail to that on the cDNA is added using terminal transferase. The two species are annealed and the recombinant molecule is held together by the hydrogen bonds between the complementary tails, as shown in Fig. 2.3. Once inside *Escherichia coli* cells the molecule is repaired and replicated.

Recently a more popular method of insertion has involved the use of DNA linkers. These are short synthetic oligonucleotides incorporating specific restriction enzyme sites. Figure 2.4 gives an example of an *Eco*R1 linker, and the cloning strategy will be illustrated using these. The oligonucleotide is self-complementary and under appropriate conditions a population of such molecules can anneal together and become double-stranded.

Linkers of this sort can be made in large quantities and thus can be ligated in their double-stranded form in vast excess to the DNA to be cloned, which is then cleaved with the restriction enzyme. Since it is possible that the DNA will already have internal *Eco*R1 sites the DNA is often treated prior to linker addition with *Eco*R1 methylase, an enzyme which adds methyl groups to the *Eco*R1 recognition sequence. This subsequently prevents cleavage at these points by the restriction enzyme. Thus the DNA is only cleaved at the linker sites. The DNA now has *Eco*R1 cohesive ends and can be inserted by ligation into an appropriate vector cleaved at a compatible site.

Alternatively, cohesive end DNA adapters can be used. These are composed of two synthetic DNA sequences which are in part complementary. However, one of the DNA species is longer than the other so that when annealing has occurred a single-stranded protrusion is produced at one end of the resulting molecule. This overhang is compatible with a restriction enzyme generated cohesive end so that ligation can occur between the two. An example of such an *Eco*R1 adapter is given in Fig. 2.5. In this case the

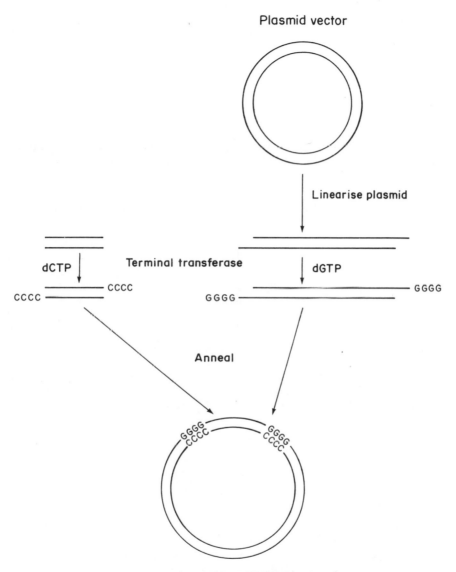

Fig. 2.3 The generation of recombinant plasmids by homopolymeric tailing. In this instance the cleaved plasmid is tailed with dGMP residues and the DNA to be inserted with dCMP molecules. Following annealing recombinant plasmids are formed

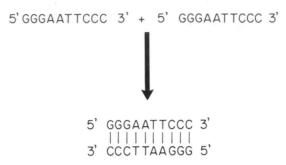

5' GGGAATTCCC 3' + 5' GGGAATTCCC 3'

5' GGGAATTCCC 3'
   | | | | | | | | | |
3' CCCTTAAGGG 5'

Fig. 2.4 An *Eco*R1 linker formed by the annealing of the synthesised oligonucleotide. The central sequence GAATTC contains the recognition site for this enzyme

5'CTTGGCGGCCGCGG 3' + 5'AATTCCGCGGCCGCCAAG 3'

5'CTTGGCGGCCGCGG 3'
  | | | | | | | | | | | | | |
3'GAACCGCCGGCGCCTTAA 5'

Fig. 2.5 An *Eco*R1 adapter formed by annealing of two synthesised oligonucleotides. The annealed molecule contains the recognition sequence for the restriction enzyme *Not*1 and the protruding end allows ligation to *Eco*R1-cleaved DNA

oligonucleotides have been designed to include the recognition sequence for the restriction enzyme *Not*1. This enzyme cuts DNA infrequently and therefore the recognition sequence is unlikely to be present in the cloned DNA. The incorporation of such a sequence in the adapter may facilitate the excision of the cloned DNA intact from the vector for subsequent analysis.

Adapters have an advantage over linkers in that when they are ligated to the DNA to be cloned a further restriction enzyme digest is not necessary. Thus internal sites do not have to be protected. The resulting DNA can be ligated directly to a suitably cleaved vector.

CLONING FROM DNA

Since DNA can be cleaved directly with restriction enzymes, the cloning procedures are much less involved than those described above for RNA. In some cases it may be sufficient to cleave the purified DNA from the organism with one restriction enzyme, followed by ligation of the resulting DNA into a vector cleaved at a compatible site. If the full genome is to be mapped, however, it may be necessary to create more than one clone bank with DNA preparations cleaved with different enzymes. Alternatively, partial digests of the DNA can be carried out so that the DNA is not cleaved at each site. Cross-hybridisation and sequencing data help to identify over-lapping clones. However, if mapping is to be carried out care must be taken in the latter method to ensure that DNA fragments from different regions of the genome do not ligate together at the ligation step. This can be achieved by treating the cleaved DNA with alkaline phosphatase, an enzyme that removes 5'-terminal phosphate groups. The resulting DNA can only be ligated to the vector which will supply 5'-phosphate groups for the reaction.

CHOICE OF VECTORS FOR CLONING

The list of vectors available for cloning has become immense. It is now pos-sible to clone into a variety of *E. coli* vectors, into yeast systems and into various mammalian vectors. The latter are important if expression is required and the protein needs to be post-translationally modified for bio-logical activity. Only the *E. coli* systems will be covered in this chapter although some of the others will be referred to later. There are three cate-gories of *E. coli* vectors which will be dealt with here.

PLASMID VECTORS

Plasmids are closed circular, double-stranded DNA molecules that repli-cate independently of the host chromosome. In early cloning experiments DNA was inserted into naturally occurring purified plasmids at suitable restriction enzyme sites. More recently, many plasmid vectors have been engineered to include a variety of desirable features to improve both the simplicity and efficiency of cloning. These include: (a) a selectable marker for cells containing the plasmid such as an antibiotic resistance gene; (b) a multiple cloning site—a short piece of DNA housing a large number of restriction enzyme sites unique for that plasmid; (c) a selection system—to differentiate between clones containing recombinant and non-recombinant plasmids. In addition such plasmids are generally small in size (2–3 kilo-bases (kb)) and, consequently, can accept up to 10 kb of foreign DNA. They generally replicate at a high copy number (up to 60 copies per bacterial cell) and can be purified readily. Following linearisation of the plasmid at one of the unique sites, foreign DNA with compatible cohesive ends can be ligated to it. Both recombinant and non-recombinant plasmids are pro-duced since the plasmid can recircularise via its own cohesive ends. This can be minimised by treatment of the plasmid with alkaline phosphatase which removes 5'-phosphate groups prior to the ligation reaction. When the ligated plasmid preparation is mixed with a suitably prepared preparation of *E. coli* cells a small proportion of cells take up plasmid molecules, a process called transformation. Such cells can be selected for by plating on agar plates containing the antibiotic, the resistance to which is encoded on the plasmid. It is necessary, however, to distinguish between colonies containing recombinant and non-recombinant plasmid molecules. Some of the earlier-used cloning plasmid vectors such as pBR322 contain two antibiotic resistance genes. Insertion of DNA into one of these inactivates that gene, and cells containing these plasmids do not survive if plated out in the presence of that antibiotic. Selection is first made on plates containing the antibiotic, the resistance gene for which is still intact. Cells containing either of the two plasmids should form colonies and these are streaked in parallel on plates each containing one of the two antibiotics. Clones containing recombinants do not grow on plates containing the antibiotic for which the gene has been inactivated. These colonies can be rescued from the other control plate, grown up and their plasmids purified for further study of the cloned DNA.

Many improved plasmid vectors, such as the pUC series of vectors, have a selection system based on the enzyme β-galactosidase. They carry a fragment containing the α-peptide coding region of this enzyme preceded by the *E. coli* lac operon promoter. Into the fifth codon of the peptide coding region has been placed a multiple cloning site (MCS). This has been achieved in such a way that a functional α-peptide is still made since the proper translational reading frame is maintained. The host *E. coli* strain used for transformation carries a defect in its β-galactosidase gene. However, this is complemented by the active peptide produced as a gene product from the plasmid, so that active β-galactosidase is produced. If cells containing these plasmids are plated on the chromogenic substrate for this enzyme, X-gal (5-bromo-4-chloro-3-indolyl-β-D-galactopyranoside), colonies will turn blue. Insertion of foreign DNA into the multiple cloning site disrupts the α-peptide coding region and complementation is not achieved. Hence cells containing such recombinant plasmids will be white when plated on X-gal. Therefore a simple blue/white selection system is achieved.

BACTERIOPHAGE λ VECTORS

The bacteriophage λ genome is approximately 50 kb long. However, only about 60% of the genome is necessary for normal lytic growth. The central part of the genome is concerned with lysogeny, a process whereby the bacteriophage inserts its genome into the host chromosome under certain conditions. All or part of this can be replaced by foreign DNA and, as a result of a process called *in vitro* packaging, lytic bacteriophage with the cloned DNA inserted in their genome can be produced. A variety of λ vectors have been generated. In some instances a simple restriction enzyme digest followed by gel electrophoresis allows the essential ends (arms) of purified genomes obtained from phage particles to be isolated and the central regions to be discarded. With certain vectors commercial preparations of such arms are available. The central region is sometimes termed a *'stuffer fragment'* and can be up to 20 kb long, and DNA of this length can be inserted. These are called λ-*replacement vectors* and are popular for genomic DNA cloning because they tolerate large inserts. In other instances bacteriophage vectors containing shortened genomes have been produced. Such vectors have been engineered to contain unique restriction sites in the central part of the genome for the insertion of foreign DNA. These are called λ-*insertion vectors*. Examples of this type of vector are λ-gt10 and λ-gt11, which are specifically useful for cDNA cloning. These contain a single *Eco*R1 site in the central part of the genome and DNA of up to 7 kb can be inserted. In addition, λ-gt11 has been designed as an expression vector and the inserted DNAs can be expressed as a β-galactosidase fusion protein. The recombinant plaques can be screened with an antibody against the protein, the coding region of which is to be isolated. *In vitro* packaging extracts are derived from λ-bacteriophage-infected bacterial cells and supply all the necessary proteins for packaging of the concatameric recombinant genomes produced in the ligation reaction. The phage used to make the extracts carry mutations which prevent their genomes being packaged. At either end of normal λ-genomes are single-stranded cohesive ends called *cos sites*. These can base-pair together to circularise the genome. However, during replication, progeny genomes are produced by a rolling circle mechanism forming a chain of linear λ-DNA molecules. An endonuclease enzyme digests this at the cos sites to produce single λ-genomes which are packaged. This enzyme is present in *in vitro* packaging extracts and cleaves the long concatameric molecules produced at the ligation step during cloning experiments at cos sites generating recombinant genomes. However, only those genomes which are at least 90% of the length of the normal genome are packaged. *In vitro* packaging results in an extremely high cloning efficiency of up to 10^8 colonies per μg DNA, which is generally better than can be achieved by plasmid cloning.

COSMID VECTORS

Cosmids are vectors into which the cos sequences from λ-bacteriophage have been inserted. These are essential for the *in vitro* packaging reaction. They generally carry an antibiotic resistance marker and a plasmid origin of replication, and therefore can replicate in *E.coli* like normal plasmids if introduced into them by transformation. They also contain unique restriction sites for linearisation. The DNA for insertion is size-selected to be between 40 and 45 kb and in the ligation reaction long concatameric molecules are generated. Those foreign DNA segments flanked by two cosmid molecules are capable of being *in vitro* packaged by packaging extracts because of the presence of the two cos sites which are cleaved during the process. Once inside the cell, cosmids assume a plasmid-like mode of replication after religation of the cos sites.

SCREENING LIBRARIES FOR THE SEQUENCE OF INTEREST

At the end of any cloning experiment it may be necessary to screen a large number of colonies/plaques to identify one containing the desired sequence. We have already seen that antibodies can be used to screen λ-gt11 expression libraries, although only one in six clones will contain inserts in the proper orientation and in the required reading frame for the production of the correct fusion protein. In this type of screening plaque impressions are made onto nylon filters which are incubated with the specific antibody. The original plates are retained. Following washing, filters are incubated with secondary anti-IgG conjugated to an enzyme and then in a chromo-genic substrate. A colour reaction denotes the position of antibody bound to plaques which are expressing the protein of interest. The corresponding plaques on the original plates can then be grown up for examination of the inserted sequence. Alternatively libraries can be screened with nucleic acid probes if they are available. These may be cloned fragments from a related species which is likely to show homology to the required sequence. If such cloned fragments are not available then it may be necessary to purify sufficient protein and to sequence it partially. From the derived amino acid sequence using reverse genetics it is possible to derive all the possible coding sequences for it. Since some amino acids have as many as six codons, care must be taken to choose a region of the protein with the corresponding minimum possible coding sequences. Oligonucleotides corresponding to these are synthesised and used as probes to select out the desired clone. Whichever method is used the nucleic acid probe sequence has to be labelled, e.g. with ^{32}P. For cloned fragments this is readily achieved by first denaturing the DNA and then carrying out a synthesis reaction on the single-stranded templates using the Klenow fragment of DNA polymerase I, random hexanucleotide primers and the four dNTPS, only one of which is labelled. It is necessary to boil the resulting DNA to make it single-stranded before it can be used as a probe. Oligonucleotides can be end-labelled using [γ-^{32}P]ATP and polynucleotide kinase. For hybridisation, impressions are made of colonies or plaques by layering a filter over them, and the trans-ferred clones are lysed and the DNA in them made single-stranded by incubating filters in NaOH. Finally the DNA is immobilised onto the filter and incubated with the single-stranded nucleic acid probe. This will seek out and bind to any cloned DNA containing the matching sequence of interest. Following washing, autoradiography is used to identify the clones to which the probe has bound.

NUCLEIC ACID SEQUENCING TECHNIQUES

A variety of methods are used to sequence nucleic acids. RNA and DNA fragments can be sequenced directly, provided that sufficient material is available. Alternatively cloned DNA fragments or polymerase chain reaction (PCR) amplified fragments are sequenced, although for longer fragments it may be necessary to sunclone into an M13 or phagemid vector. The two principal methods are the chemical degradation procedure of Maxam and Gilbert (1977) and the di-deoxynucleotide nucleotide chain termination method developed by Sangar and Coulson (1975). Both methods rely on the ability to separate nucleic acid sequences differing by only one nucleotide in length on denaturing polyacrylamide gels.

CHEMICAL DEGRADATION METHOD

The most common starting material for this method of sequencing is a specific cloned fragment from the region of interest. In order to provide a reference point and to facilitate autoradiography of the final gel, the fragment is generally end-labelled with a radioactive residue (either ^{32}P or ^{35}S). Polynucleotide kinase and [γ-^{32}P]ATP can be used to label the 5′ ends, provided the restriction fragment has previously been treated with alkaline phosphatase. Alternatively the 3′ ends can be labelled using terminal deoxynucleotidyl transferase and [α-^{32}P]cordycepin or di-deoxynucleotide ATP as substrate. It may also be possible to fill in ends using the Klenow fragment of DNA polymerase I if 5′ protruding ends have been left by the restriction enzymes. Should the fragments have been created by two restriction enzymes, one leaving a 5′ and the other a 3′ protruding end, then it is possible to use the fill-in reaction to label only one end of the fragment. Most of the other methods result in both ends being labelled, and steps have to be taken to produce a fragment with a single label. This is achieved by either cleaving the fragment asymmetrically at an internal restriction site and retrieving each of the smaller fragments from a suitable gel or by denaturing the fragment to achieve strand separation and again recovering the separated strands using gel electrophoresis. The DNA species thus generated is next divided and each portion is subjected to a different chemical treatment designed to modify the molecule specifically at positions of one or in some cases two of the four nucleotides. Strand scission is generally completed using piperidine in each case. The modification treatment is adjusted so that reactions are only partial and random with ideally, on average, only one nucleotide affected per DNA molecule. There have been many DNA modification reactions described but only four of the most commonly used are described briefly here. Methylation of guanine at the N-7 position and adenine at the N-3 position is achieved using dimethylsulphate. Subsequent treatment with alkaline piperidine specifically causes displacement of the ring-opened G, and removal of

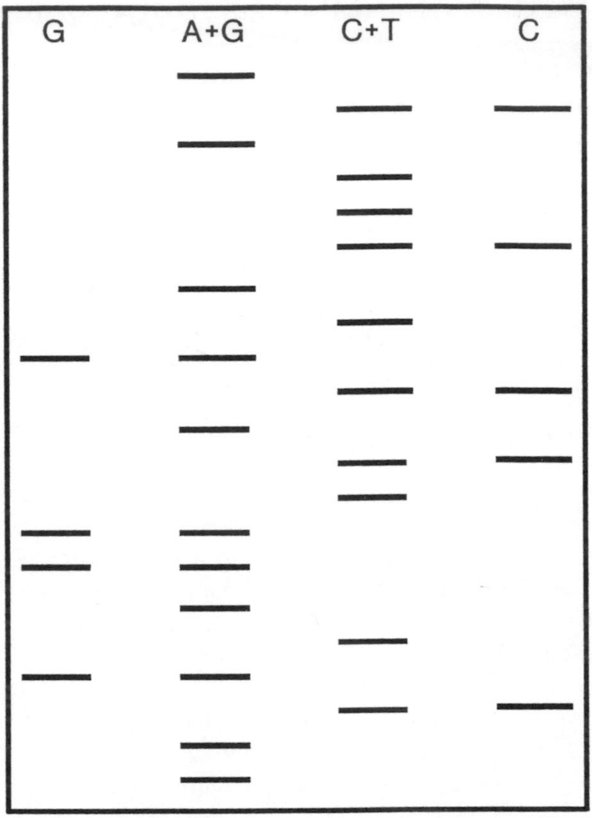

Fig. 2.6 Diagrammatic representation of the banding pattern obtained when the 5′ end labelled oligonucleotide 5′-AACGTAGGTCACGTACTTGCA-3′ is sequenced using the chemical degradation procedures described in the text

flanking phosphates leads to strand cleavage. Cleavage at both A and G residues following methylation can be achieved using mild acid conditions. Treatment with hydrazine modifies pyrimidine residues, which again can be displaced by piperidine followed by strand breakage. However, the presence of salt in the modification reaction causes suppression of the thymine reaction and thus gives rise to a cytosine-specific reaction. At the end of the chemical degradation procedure each reaction mix should contain a population of molecules of varying length depending on the position at which the specified strand cleavage has occurred. A proportion of these will be end-labelled with ^{32}P and these can be visualised by autoradiography following separation on the basis of size using denaturing polyacrylamide gel electrophoresis. The four reactions are run in adjacent lanes of the gel, and after autoradiography the consecutive shift of the label to the various lanes allows the deduction of the nucleotide sequence from the labelled end. A diagrammatic profile of the banding pattern obtained from the sequence 5'-AACGTAGGTCACGTACTTGCA-3', end-labelled with ^{32}P, is shown in Fig. 2.6.

Today, the chemical degradation method is not used as widely as the chain terminator method but is useful in specific instances.

THE DI-DEOXYNUCLEOTIDE NUCLEOTIDE CHAIN TERMINATION METHOD

This method has become the most common of the two procedures because of its greater versatility, quickness and higher accuracy. It depends on the controlled interruption of DNA synthesis, starting from a specific primer annealed to the nucleic acid species to be sequenced. This can be single-stranded RNA, single-stranded DNA or denatured double-stranded DNA, and various DNA polymerases such as reverse transcriptase, the Klenow fragment of *E. coli* DNA polymerase 1, λ- bacteriophage T7 DNA polymerase or *Thermus aquaticus* (Taq) DNA polymerase can be used for the synthesis reaction. In this case it is the primer annealing position that acts as the reference point. Thus to ensure that the primer anneals accurately it is usually about 17–24 nucleotides long.

The normal substrates for DNA synthesis are the four deoxynucleotide triphosphates dATP, dCTP, dGTP and dTTP (dNTPs). If the primer is annealed to the template and added to the dNTPs and a DNA polymerase under the appropriate conditions, chain extension will occur from the 3'-OH group of the primer with a complementary copy of the template being made. Controlled interruption of this synthesis can be achieved by incorporating an analogue of one of the dNTPs in the reaction. The most common analogues to be used are the di-deoxynucleotide nucleotide triphosphates (ddNTP), the structures of which are illustrated in Fig. 2.7 and compared with the normal substrate dNTP.

These can be incorporated into a growing DNA chain like an ordinary dNTP, but because they lack a 3'-OH group a phosphodiester cannot be formed between them and the next incoming nucleotide, and thus chain termination occurs. However, if one of the dNTPs is completely replaced by its corresponding analogue in the synthesis reaction, chain termination would always occur at the first site of incorporation of that ddNTP giving only a single complementary DNA species of defined length. Thus an appropriate mixture of dNTPs and ddNTPs is used so that only partial incorporation of the ddNTP occurs at each possible site, resulting at the end of the synthesis in a mixture of DNA molecules complementary to the template and each ending with the ddNTP included in the reaction. The length of each resulting strand is therefore determined by the position of the complementary nucleotide in the template relative to the primer. For complete sequencing the primed DNA is divided into four separate reactions. Each

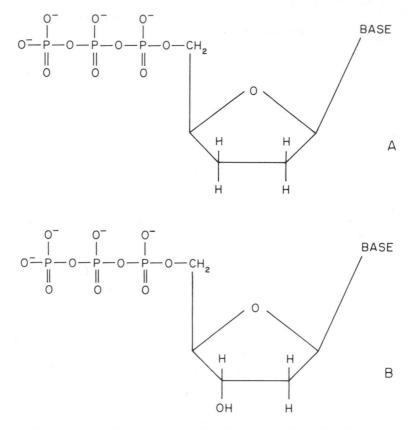

Fig. 2.7 The structure of a di-deoxynucleotide triphosphate (A). The structure of the normal deoxynucleotide triphosphate is shown for comparison (B)

reaction has the four normal dNTPs added, one of which may be radioactively labelled to enable visualisation of the bands following gel electrophoresis. In addition, to each reaction is added a different ddNTP. Following chain extension from the primer, the reactions are boiled in a denaturing solution to release the newly synthesised complementary DNA molecules from their templates, and these are then electrophoresed on adjacent lanes of a polyacrylamide gel. Following autoradiography it is possible to read the sequence of the complementary molecules by observing the position of the bands from the bottom of the gel.

CLONING VECTORS FOR DI-DEOXYNUCLEOTIDE NUCLEOTIDE SEQUENCING

One of the essential features of di-deoxynucleotide sequencing is that part of the template sequence must be known so that a primer can be synthesised that will anneal accurately to it. To sequence a large piece of DNA directly, primers would have to be made at 200–300 base-pair intervals, which is the resolving power of most gels. To circumvent this problem, in most large-scale sequencing projects the DNA is subcloned after suitable enzyme treatment into M13 or phagemid cloning vectors. M13 is an *E. coli* bacteriophage which has a single-stranded circular genome of approximately 7.5 kb, designated the plus strand. In infected cells, the M13 genome is converted into a double-stranded molecule by host cell enzymes which synthesise a complementary or minus stranded copy. This double-stranded DNA is called the replicative form or RF. The positive strand is nicked by a viral gene product, and *E. coli* DNA polymerase I extends from the new 3' end, displacing the original strand. This is called the rolling circle mode of replication. Once each circle of replication is complete another virus-encoded protein cleaves the new positive strands to generate progeny viral-length genomes which are then ligated into circles. These are used as templates to produce further RF molecules in the early stages of infection but later are packaged by coat proteins to produce progeny particles which are extruded into the medium without lysing the *E. coli* cells. Late in infection there can be as many as 100–200 RF molecules in each *E. coli* cell, and it is possible to purify these using standard plasmid isolation techniques. It is also possible to initiate an infection by transforming *E. coli* cells with RF molecules. Progeny M13 particles are produced from transformants which infect neighbouring cells. However, the growth of such cells is retarded compared with cells that are not infected. Thus, if a mixture of both types of cell are mixed with agar and plated out, small plaques are formed, each arising initially from a single cell which has taken up an RF molecule. Such RF molecules have been genetically engineered to include the α-peptide coding region of β-galactosidase (amino acids 1–45) inserted between genes II and IV of the phage. A series of vectors have been created by inserting a number of unique restriction enzyme sites in the N-terminal region of the α-peptide, thus providing a cluster of different multiple cloning sites. These have been inserted such that the reading frame is maintained. These RF molecules are still capable of establishing an infection following transformation of *E. coli* cells. A strain of host cells is used which carries a defect in its β-galactosidase gene. However, this is complemented by the α-peptide produced in cells transformed by vector RF molecules yielding active β-galactosidase. If cells are plated on, the chromogenic substrate (X-gal) and an inducer for the enzyme blue plaques are formed. It is possible to clone up to 1 kb of foreign DNA into the multiple cloning site of the RF molecules of such vectors and, again, to use standard transformation techniques to insert the recombinant molecules back into *E. coli*. The inserted DNA fragment normally disrupts the α-peptide sequence, resulting in a loss of β-galactosidase activity, thus recombinant phage plaques are clear. Consequently a direct selection of plaques containing cells which are likely to contain phage with inserts can be made. Such plaques can be picked individually and grown in liquid culture. The RF molecules in infected cells are used to produce progeny single-stranded DNA genomes each containing cloned DNA. These genomes are packaged and the mature bacteriophage is extruded into the medium without causing lysis of the bacterial cell. After centrifugation to pellet the cells the bacteriophage can be concentrated and their genomes obtained by phenol extraction. Being single-stranded they act as perfect templates for di-deoxynucleotide nucleotide sequencing. The primer used is chosen to anneal to a region of the M13 part of the molecule just outside the 3' end of the multiple cloning site. Such a primer can be used to sequence across any fragment inserted at the chosen site using the protocols described above.

The use of M13 for sequencing has been widespread and extremely useful. However, because of the relative instability of the genome and the fact that usually only up to 1 kb can be cloned into the RF, it is rarely used as an initial cloning vector. Generally, fragments are subcloned into it prior to sequencing. To circumvent this task a number of vectors have been developed called *phagemids* which contain some desirable features of both plasmids and filamentous bacteriophages. They contain a plasmid origin of replication, a selectable marker such as an antibiotic resistance gene and multiple cloning sites. They are generally small in size and can accommodate up to 10 kb of foreign DNA. Vectors into which foreign DNA has been cloned can be propagated as normal plasmids. However, the vector also contains the major intergenic region of a filamentous bacteriophage such as M13 or f1. This region contains the sequences necessary for phage DNA synthesis and for genome packaging. When infected with helper phage, cells containing the phagemid switch from the plasmid replication mode to a rolling circle mode so that single-stranded DNA containing the cloned sequence is produced. This DNA is packaged and extruded from cells in the form of bacteriophage particles. It can be purified and used as templates for DNA sequencing, as described above, using a primer which anneals to a sequence beside the multiple cloning site.

POLYMERASE CHAIN REACTION (PCR)

The recent advances in gene amplification methods have greatly facilitated the accumulation of sequencing data. The method used is the PCR, which allows amplification of specific fragments of DNA provided that sequences flanking the required region are known. This eliminates the need to make and screen full clone banks in many cases in order to obtain a clone containing the sequence of interest. Primers corresponding to the flanking regions are synthesised and incubated with DNA containing the target sequence, dNTPs and *Thermus aquaticus* DNA polymerase I (Taq polymerase), an enzyme that is very thermostable. The reaction mixture is cycled through a series of temperature steps. The DNA is denatured (i.e. made single-stranded) by heating it at 95°C, the reaction mixture is cooled to 55°C to allow the primer to anneal to its target sequence, and primer extension is carried out at the temperature optimum for the enzyme, i.e. 72°C, thus generating further copies of the required sequence. Each cycle lasts less than 12 minutes. On further cycles of heat denaturation and synthesis the yields of the target fragment rise exponentially, and generally 30–40 cycles are enough to allow visualisation of a portion of the product following gel electrophoresis. The process is shown diagrammatically in Fig. 2.8.

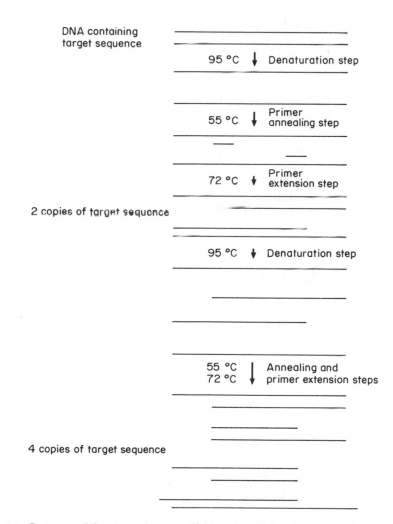

Fig. 2.8 Gene amplification of target DNA using the polymerase chain reaction. Each cycle involves a DNA denaturation step, followed by a primer-annealing step and finally a primer extension step. Only two cycles are illustrated, resulting in four copies of the target sequence. Each subsequent cycle will double the number of copies

Many variations of the method have been developed. For example, primers have been designed which incorporate restriction enzyme sites at their 5′ ends to facilitate subsequent cloning of the generated fragments. RNA, too, can be used as a starting material provided that a reverse transcriptase step is first carried out. The cDNA that is produced acts as a template for gene amplification. Following purification, fragments can be sequenced directly using a modification of the chain terminator sequencing method described above. Alternatively they can be cloned into DNA sequencing vectors for sequence determination.

SUMMARY

The elucidation of the sequence of the cloned gene is only a starting point for the determination of epitopes. As previously mentioned, sequence comparisons between strains of viruses may indicate variable regions which potentially are important B-cell epitopes. The sequencing of monoclonal antibody escape mutants has in many instances indicated the residues that contribute to such sites. Computer programs are available that can determine from the sequence where there are possible T-cell epitopes. In Chapters 3 and 4 the application of information on gene sequences to the elucidation of the amino acids that constitute important epitope sites is more fully explained.

SUGGESTED READING

Maxam AM and Gilbert W (1979) A new method for sequencing DNA. *Proc. Natl Acad. Sci. USA.* **74**, 560–564.

Sangar F and Coulson AR (1975) A rapid method for determining sequences in DNA by primed synthesis with DNA polymerase. *J. Mol. Biol.* **94**, 441–448.

Watson JD , Witkowski J, Gilman M and Zoller M (1992) *Recombinant DNA.* Scientific American Books. W.H. Freeman & Co.

3 Requirements for the Induction of Immunity

INTRODUCTION

In the previous chapter we have seen how recombinant DNA technology can be used to define the nucleic acid sequence of the genes coding for the proteins of infectious agents. In order to make full use of this information for the design of vaccines, it is necessary to understand how the immune system reacts to invading organisms. The immune system responds to antigens. The parts of the antigens recognised are termed T- and B-cell epitopes. We need to understand how such epitopes are recognised and what are the parameters that control their immunogenicity. This chapter will outline the processes leading to the production of an immune response in terms of the requirements for immunogenicity and the cell types involved. A starting point is to consider the ways our potential vaccine will differ from the pathogen and how this may affect the immune response to it.

THE VACCINE CONCEPT

An ideal vaccine may be considered to be a modified, non-pathogenic form of an infectious agent, not as capable of replication and spread as the wild type or pathogenic agent, but still able to stimulate the immune system. Indeed some of our best vaccines, such as the Sabin polio vaccine, differ only slightly from their parental disease-causing organism and yet portray a lack of pathogenicity. By following the same route of infection as poliovirus, i.e. the gastrointestinal tract, the live-attenuated vaccine encounters the same defence systems and cells as the pathogenic virus and thus stimulates them to respond in a manner similar to that seen in a natural infection. Unfortunately, it is not always possible to develop such vaccines for all viral, bacterial or parasitic pathogens. One alternative is to use killed organisms as vaccines, but these, while useful in the short term, often fail to induce long-lasting immunity. To induce immunity to many microbial agents and all eukaryotic parasites it is necessary to use vaccines based on a subunit of the organism. Such subunits will be unlikely to contain the elements needed for independent infection, multiplication or growth in the host. For the purposes of this book we will use the term *live vaccine* for those agents that can replicate and multiply, while the term *dead vaccine* will be used for preparations which are unable to replicate, including inactivated, killed, subunits or synthetic material.

We will now try and explain as fully as possible the events which under-lie the initiation of the immune response and identify the components of the immune system which are required to be stimulated in order to induce resistance to infection. In understanding these events, we may be able not only to maximise these processes but also to avoid the induction of responses which might increase or alter pathogenesis on subsequent expos-ure to infection, which can be a major problem in vaccination programmes.

ROUTES OF ENTRY INTO THE BODY

Infectious agents may enter the body by a variety of routes; these include through the skin, gastric epithelia, the lungs and by direct inoculation such as by insect bites. The route of entry to the body determines to some degree which components of the immune system will be the first to respond to the infectious agent. Although much of the effector system and all of the mem-ory of the immune system resides in the clonal expansion of various types of lymphocyte populations, the full expression of the activity of these cells is dependent, in the majority of cases, on interaction with a diverse group of cell types known collectively by their functional title of *antigen-presenting cells* (APC). It is these cells which provide the initial interaction between an antigen and the adaptive immune system. APCs process and present anti-gens to lymphocytes—the cells in which the memory function of the immune response resides. Lymphocytes, like other leucocytes, are initially produced in the bone marrow but then differentiate along two separate pathways. Those which undergo a period of development and differentiation in the *thymus* are known as T-cells and are involved mainly in cell-to-cell interac-tions such as augmentation of immune responses ($CD4^+$ helper T-cells), sup-pression of immune responses ($CD8^+$ suppressor T-cells) or the secretion of *cytokines*. Those cells which are not influenced by the thymic environment are known as B-cells and differentiate into cells which produce antibodies. Lymphocytes form the basis of both the memory required for successful vaccination and a major part of the effector arm of the immune response.

CHARACTERISTICS AND LOCATION OF ANTIGEN-PRESENTING CELLS

Table 3.1 compares some APCs which are capable of presenting antigen to helper T-lymphocytes and thus initiating an anamnestic (memory) immune response. The Langerhans cells of the skin circulate between the dermis and the relevant draining lymph nodes (where they become follicular dendritic

Table 3.1 Characteristics of antigen-presenting cells

	Location	MHC Class II	Phagocytic	Recirculating
Langerhans	Skin	+	−	+
Macrophage	Tissues	+	+	−
Activated B-lymphocyte	Lymph nodes	+	−	?

cells). One can see that, although phagocytosis is not a prerequisite for antigen presentation, the expression of *MHC class II molecules* on the cell surface is necessary.

THE MAJOR HISTOCOMPATIBILITY COMPLEX AND IMMUNOGENICITY

A considerable amount is now known about the genetics of the major histocompatibility complex (MHC) system. In humans the genes which code for the products of the MHC are found on chromosome 6, whereas a similar group of genes are located on chromosome 17 in mice. The H2 region in the mouse and the HLA region in man code for a range of polypeptides which are classified as classes I, II or III MHC molecules.

Class I is made up of the histocompatibility antigens found on all nucleated cells (mouse regions K, D and Qa; human regions HLA-A, B, C). T-Lymphocytes bearing the CD8 antigen, that is to say suppressor/cytotoxic cells, recognise antigen in association with the class I molecule. As such they may form part of the immune response induced by a vaccine. Similarly class III molecules encode complement components which increase the effectiveness of both innate and adaptive immune responses. It is, however, the class II molecules which are central to immunogenicity in that they determine which parts of an antigen can serve as epitopes. As noted above, cells bearing class II molecules (mouse Ia, human HLA-D) are required for presentation of antigen to helper (CD4$^+$) T-cells. There is considerable genetic polymorphism within the MHC region, and as expression of MHC genes is co-dominant in an outbred population both parental molecules will be present. Biochemical and biophysical studies on class II molecules have indicated that they are composed of an α- and β-chain, and that the antigen-binding region is a cleft formed by an eight-strand β-pleated sheet supporting two helical segments. Although the class II molecules generally are polymorphic, the antigen-binding region appears to be strictly conserved for each allele but varies between alleles. This means an individual can have at most only two types of class II molecules to bind all antigens. One can compare this to the situation with other antigen-binding molecules such as immunoglobulin or the T-cell receptor (TCR) where an infinite number of antigen-combining sites can be generated by multiple genes, genetic rearrangements and somatic mutations. The revelation of the structure of MHC molecules has prompted a search for the common structural features of peptides able to combine with them. Grey and colleagues have examined a number of antigenic polypeptides which bind to the mouse class II molecule Ia^d and by use of synthetic peptides have defined the core region in each which is involved in MHC binding. These are shown in Table 3.2.

Table 3.2 Ia^d binding: a common motif

Peptide		Residue no.					
		1	2	3	4	5	6
OVA	327–332	Val	His	Ala	Ala	His	Ala
HA	135–140	Val	Thr	Ala	Ala	Lys	Ser
MYO	66–71	Val	Thr	Val	Leu	Thr	Ala
MYO	112–117	Ile	His	Val	Leu	His	Ser
Nase	104–109	Val	Arg	Gln	Gly	Leu	Ala
Nase	15–20	Ile	Lys	Ala	Ile	Asp	Gly

Key: OVA, ovalbumin; HA, influenza haemagglutinin; MYO, sperm whale myoglobulin; Nase, staphylococcal nuclease.

A common structural motif appears to be a hexapeptide which contains a hydrophobic residue at position 1, a basic or polar residue at position 2, hydrophobic residues at positions 3 and 4, variable residues at position 5 and residues with either short or no side chains at position 6.

By utilising synthetic peptides with either conservative or non-conservative substitutions it has been possible to determine which residues are involved in binding to the MHC cleft. For example, the haemagglutinin of influenza has a duodecapeptide (HA residues 307–319) which is able to stimulate a response *in vitro* by HA-specific T-cell clones when presented on cells bearing HLA-DR1. The peptide must thus be combining with both the HLA-DR and TCR molecules. As a result of experiments in which each residue was tested for its availability to an additional ligand after association with a HLA-DR molecule, Grey proposed the model shown in Fig. 3.1 in which the class II molecule and TCR binding residues lie on opposite sides of an α-helix. In fact, many T-cell epitopes are amphipathic (having hydrophobic and hydrophilic residues segregated on opposite sides of the helix).

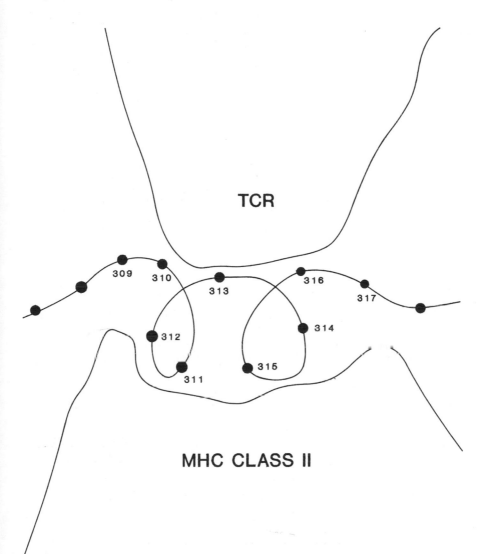

Fig. 3.1 Interaction between T-cell receptor, antigen and class II molecules

The concept of an amphipathic helix as being important in binding to the TCR has been supported by several other experimental studies, and computer programs are available which can scan sequence data for motifs associated with immunogenicity and thus highlight areas of a molecule with potential for incorporation into a subunit vaccine.

From the preceding discussion it will be apparent that those parts of a molecule which can interact with APCs are limited to those regions exhibiting certain structures. The association of the immunogen with the class II MHC molecule is preceded by its partial digestion, either internally or on the cell surface, by the proteolytic enzymes of the APC. This has the effect of reducing still further the regions of the antigen molecule which participate in the interaction with the APC and T-cell.

THE DIRECTION OF THE IMMUNE RESPONSE BY ANTIGEN-PRESENTING CELLS

The different types of APC (Table 3.1) may influence the efficiency of presentation of the antigens they bind. Thus macrophages can phagocytose bacteria and break them down in lysosomal vacuoles, producing digested fragments which are then transported to the cell membrane for presentation in association with the MHC class II molecules. It can be envisaged that this provides a system more able to process complex antigens than the *Langerhans cell*, which, being non-phagocytic, must rely on membrane-associated peptidases for the processing of antigen. In an analogous manner it is possible that class II MHC molecule bearing B-lymphocytes may provide a means of dealing with soluble antigens which are present at limiting concentrations in the micro-environment. As they carry an antigen-specific receptor (immunoglobulin) in their cell membranes this may serve to concentrate antigen prior to association with MHC molecules. As with other non-phagocytic APCs the proteolytic digestion of the antigen will be limited to that carried out by the peptidases present on the cell membrane.

The subset of APC initiating an immune response determines not only the level of immunogenicity but also the type of cells involved in the resulting effector arm of the process. As the same region of a molecule may react with both the APC and a helper T-cell as shown in Fig. 3.1, the constraints imposed by serving as a ligand for an MHC molecule may also determine the subset of helper T-cells recruited to the response. Studies on rodents have indicated that there are at least two functional subsets of helper T-cells. These differ in the range of cytokines they secrete and hence influence the involvement of other immune effector cells. In addition to certain common cytokines secreted by both subclasses, T-helper 1 (T_H1) cells secrete interleukin 2 (IL-2), γ interferon (IFNγ) and lymphotoxin (LT), all of which activate inflammatory cells. On the other hand, T-helper 2 (T_H2) cells characteristically produce interleukins 4, 5, 6 and 10. IL-4, IL-5 and IL-6 are involved in the growth and differentiation of B-lymphocytes, while IL-10 is thought to down-regulate the activity of T_H1 cells. These reactions are shown schematically in Fig. 3.2.

Different types of APC appear to exhibit a preference in the subclass of T-helper cell with which they interact. For example, liver macrophages (Kupfer cells) interact only with T_H1 cells.

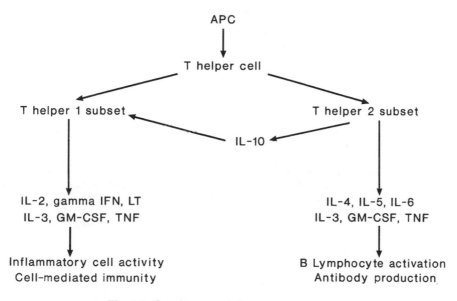

Fig. 3.2 Cytokines and the immune response

In many infections the presence of a variety of epitopes at several sites in the body will result in both subclasses of T_H cell being activated, producing an immune response which has both humoral and cell-mediated effector systems. Where B-cells are involved in the ensuing immune response then epitopes capable of being bound by specific immunoglobulin must be accessible. It is becoming evident that in many cases resistance to reinfection may depend on a specific response, others being either irrelevant or deleterious. For example, immunity to mycobacterial infections is wholly dependent on the presence of activated macrophages, a T_H1-dependent reaction, while stimulation of T_H2 cells reduces the effectiveness of this reaction through the action of IL-10. It is thus essential when designing subunit vaccines that those components of the immunogen which will stimulate the T_H subset required for a protective immune response are determined.

SUMMARY

The induction of an anamnestic immune response requires the involvement of T-lymphocytes. Antigens are recognised by T-helper lymphocytes in the context of the MHC class II molecule, leading to genetically based differences in immune responsiveness. The MHC class II bearing cell with which the T-cell interacts may also determine the balance of effector cells and molecules produced in the subsequent immune response. If resistance to infection is dependent on the production of antibody then the immunogen incorporated in the subunit vaccine must include a region which can act as a ligand for immunoglobulin, that is, a B-cell epitope, in addition to the regions capable of binding to the APC and TCR.

SUGGESTED READING

Braciale TJ and Braciale VL (1991) Antigen presentation: Structural themes and functional variations. *Immunology Today* **12**(4), 124–129.
Mosman TR and Moore KW (1991) The role of IL-10 in cross-regulation of Th1 and Th2 responses. *Immunology Today* **12**(3), 49–53.

4 Prediction of Epitopes

INTRODUCTION

In Chapter 2 we have indicated how the nucleotide sequence of parts of the genome of viruses, bacteria and parasites and their transcripts may be determined. From these sequences of nucleic acids, it is a relatively small step to determine the amino acid sequence of the protein that the genes encode by searching for open reading frames (ORFs). ORFs start with an AUG triplet encoding methionine, and often it is fairly easy to determine whether a particular AUG encodes the first methionine residue in a protein from the sequence context in which it is found. A set of rules has been developed which allows definition of the consensus sequences surrounding such a codon as CCRCCAUGG (where R=purine, A or G). The prediction that a particular codon signifies the start of a protein may be verified if sufficient amounts of the antigenic protein can be isolated to sequence the N-terminal amino acid residues directly. Provided that the genes that encode a particular antigenic protein do not have too complex a splicing pattern or that cDNA clones are available which have been derived from mature mRNA, it may be possible to determine the primary amino acid sequence of an antigenic protein.

Further complications in determining the primary structure of translation products result from processes which alter the translation of particular messenger RNAs. For example, it has recently been discovered that the expression of a number of viral and bacterial proteins require the ribosome to shift from one translational reading frame into another. Other examples have been described in which ribosomes jump over stretches of untranslated nucleotides within the sequence of an mRNA molecule. The discovery that RNA molecules can be edited post-transcriptionally provides a further problem in the direct 'translation' of a DNA sequence into primary protein structure.

In this chapter we will examine the procedures that allow the prediction and identification of both B-cell and T-cell epitopes, based on knowledge of the primary amino acid sequence of the antigenic protein. Unfortunately, as yet, predictive methods for carbohydrates and other macromolecular structures associated with foreign invaders have not been developed.

B-CELL EPITOPES

In order to design subunit vaccines we must know the immunogenic regions of the proteins. Such regions can be formed from contiguous stretches of primary amino acid sequences in the case of so-called *linear epitopes* or they can consist on non-contiguous stretches of amino acid residues that are brought together by the folding of the chain of amino acids of one or more proteins into *conformational epitopes*. The latter cannot be predicted from primary sequence data only and their verification requires other techniques, outlined towards the end of this chapter. For the prediction of linear epitopes in proteins a number of computer programs have been developed. They analyse both characteristics of the linear sequences as well as make predictions about the secondary structure of the proteins.

HYDROPHOBICITY AND HYDROPHILICITY

Linear characteristics such as the summation of the hydrophilicity or hydrophobicity of particular amino acids can be determined for a small number of residues and plotted as a running average. Two methods are used: that of Kyte and Doolittle (1982), which sums up the *hydropathy* (hydrophobicity) values of residues; and that of Hopp and Woods (1981), which originally was described as a measure of the antigenicity of a given sequence but is based on the sum of the hydrophilicity of a number of residues. The difference between these methods lies in the relative values of hydrophobicity and hydrophilicity assigned to each of the amino acid residues. These have been determined from the positions of amino acid residues in protein sequences from which the tertiary structure is also known (see Table 4.1). The hydrophobicity values in the Kyte and Doolittle scale are positive for

Table 4.1 Hydrophilicity and hydrophobicity values of amino acid residues in proteins

Residue		KD value	HW value	Residue		KD value	HW value
pro	P	−1.6	0	ser	S	−0.8	0.3
gly	G	−0.4	0	thr	T	−0.7	−0.4
val	V	4.2	−1.5	glu	E	−3.5	3.0
ile	I	4.5	−1.8	asp	D	−3.0	3.0
leu	L	3.8	−1.8	his	H	−3.2	−0.5
ala	A	1.8	−0.5	lys	K	−3.9	3.0
met	M	1.9	−1.3	arg	R	−4.5	3.0
gln	Q	−3.5	0.2	phe	F	2.8	−2.5
asn	N	−3.5	0.2	tyr	Y	−1.3	−2.3
cys	C	2.5	−1.0	trp	W	−0.9	−3.4

KD hydrophobicity values as determined by Kyte and Doolittle are positive for hydrophobic residues (e.g. tryptophan), and HW hydrophilicity values as determined by Hopp and Woods are positive for hydrophilic residues (e.g. aspartic acid).

the hydrophobic amino acids, while in the Hopp and Woods scale the most hydrophilic residues attract the more positive values as the hydrophilic residues were considered most likely to be antigenic. The length of the window, i.e. the number of residues over which the summation is calculated, is adjustable, but most frequently the values of between 8 and 12 residues are summated.

SURFACE PROBABILITY AND FLEXIBILITY

Other programs that determine some characteristic of primary protein sequences by summation are those used for the determination of the surface probability and the flexibility of a particular sequence of amino acids. The surface probability index calculates the chance that a particular stretch of amino acids is localised on the surface of the protein. The flexibility of a particular stretch of amino acid residues can be calculated on the basis of the flexibilities of known residues in proteins for which the structure has been determined.

A program to estimate the probability that a given sequence of amino acids is on the surface has been developed by Emini and colleagues (1985) and is based on the calculation for a given point (residue n) in the sequence of the normalised product of the surface probabilities of amino acids in positions $n-2$ to $n+3$ in the sequence. On the basis of the crystal structure of 28 proteins, Janin and his colleagues (1978) determined the fractional probabilities that a given residue is at the surface of a protein. In order to be defined as being on the surface a residue had to have more than 2 nm^2 of its surface accessible to water. These fractional probabilities range from 0.26 for cysteine to 0.97 for lysine. The surface probability, which is the product of the six fractional probabilities of the residue in positions $n-2$ to $n+3$, is then calculated. Thus for a stretch of six cysteine residues the surface probability would be $(0.26)^6 = 0.0003089$ and for six residues of lysine it would be $(0.97)^6 = 0.8329$. The logarithm of the surface probability is then determined for each position in the protein (respectively -3.5101 for a stretch of six cysteine residues and -0.07937 for a stretch of six lysine residues). These are normalised for the whole sequence, so that a random hexapeptide has a surface probability of 1.0. After normalisation the values are plotted for each position in the amino acid sequence. Values greater than one then indicate a peptide sequence that is more likely to be at the surface of the protein than the rest of the protein, and values below one are indicative of peptide sequences most likely to occur on the inside of the protein.

The flexibility of a particular stretch of an amino acid sequence has again been calculated from data derived from X-ray crystallographic analysis of proteins. Karplus and Schulz (1985) analysed 31 protein structures which had been refined with temperature factors—a measure of the flexibility of a particular residue. They used the temperature factors (B values) for the α carbons of all the residues in the proteins included in their analysis, excluding the three at the N- and C-termini. The latter are known to have a high level of flexibility and are also known to be often very antigenic. The average value was then established for each amino acid and normalized to produce an average value (B_{norm}) of 1.000 for all 20 amino acids. The B_{norm} values rank the amino acids in decreasing order of flexibility as K (B_{norm} = 1.193; flexible), S, G, P, D, E, Q, T, N, R, A, L, H, V, Y, I, F, C, W, M (B_{norm} = 0.925; rigid). The B values for each type of amino acid residue were further refined by looking at the B values of a particular amino acid when it was flanked by one or two rigid residues. These were defined as residues with a flexibility of less than 1.000 (i.e. A, L, H, V, Y, I, F, C, W, M) in the protein structures that made up the data set from which the values were calculated. For example, the B_{norm} value for serine drops from 1.169 to 1.048 when flanked by one 'rigid' residue (i.e. a residue with a low flexibility value) to 0.923 when flanked by two 'rigid' residues. These latter values are referred to as the neighbour-correlated B_{norm} values, and these are used to establish the relative flexibility in any position of a protein in which we wish to predict linear epitopes. The relative flexibility at a position n in the sequence is calculated as the weighted sum of the neighbour-correlated B_{norm} values at positions $n-3$, $n-2$, $n-1$, n, $n+1$, $n+2$ and $n+3$ using the weights of 0.25, 0.50, 0.75, 1.00, 0.75, 0.50 and 0.25, respectively. An example of this calculation and the influence of replacement of one residue by one other is given in Table 4.2.

Table 4.2 Determination of chain flexibility of a peptide sequence

Peptide sequence	Peptide sequence								
	H	**F**	**Q**	**G**	**S**	**Y**	**D**	**C**	**W**
No rigid neighbour	0.982	0.930	1.165	**1.142**	1.169	**0.961**	1.033	0.960	0.925
One rigid neighbour	0.952	**0.912**	**1.028**	1.042	**1.048**	0.930	1.089	**0.878**	0.917
Two rigid neighbours	0.894	0.914	0.885	0.923	0.923	0.837	**0.932**	0.925	0.803
Value of position		0.25	0.50	0.75	1.00	0.75	0.50	0.25	

Corrected B_{norm} value at S:
  $0.25 \times 0.912 + 0.50 \times 1.028 + 0.75 \times 1.142 + 1.00 \times 1.048 + 0.75 \times 0.961 + 0.50 \times 0.932 + 0.25 \times 0.878 = 4.033:4$
  $= 1.008$.

If we changed the Y residue to another D the corrected B_{norm} value at S would become:
  $0.25 \times 0.912 + 0.50 \times 1.028 + 0.75 \times 1.142 + 1.00 \times 1.169 + 0.75 \times 1.033 + 0.50 \times 1.033 + 0.25 \times 0.875 = 4.277:4$
  $= 1.069$.

The B_{norm} values are determined by Karplus and Schulz. The flexibility of a given peptide sequence HFQGSYDCW is calculated for the position of the serine residue. 'Rigid' amino acids in the sequence are printed in bold. The B_{norm} value chosen on the basis of the rigidity of neighbouring amino acid residues are also printed in bold. Replacement of the Y residue by another D residue changes the flexibility calculated for the position of the S residue (affected figures are printed in italics).

SECONDARY STRUCTURE PREDICTIONS

The above methods are based on calculations of a parameter of a part of the primary sequence. Secondary structure prediction algorithms have also been developed. For many proteins not enough purified material is

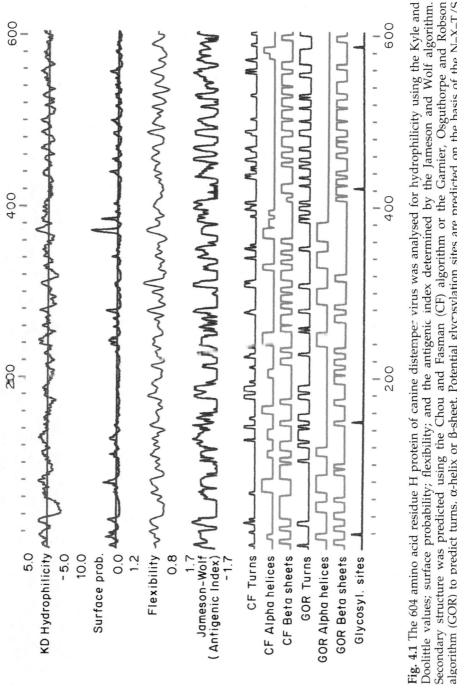

Fig. 4.1 The 604 amino acid residue H protein of canine distemper virus was analysed for hydrophilicity using the Kyle and Doolittle values; surface probability; flexibility; and the antigenic index determined by the Jameson and Wolf algorithm. Secondary structure was predicted using the Chou and Fasman (CF) algorithm or the Garnier, Osguthorpe and Robson algorithm (GOR) to predict turns, α-helix or β-sheet. Potential glycosylation sites are predicted on the basis of the N–X–T/S motif

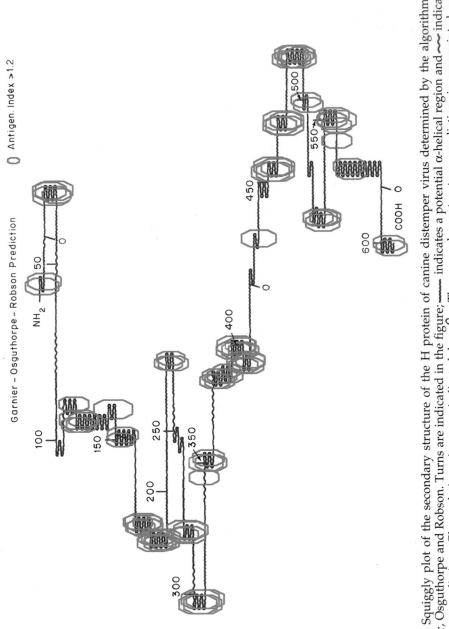

Fig 4.2 Squiggly plot of the secondary structure of the H protein of canine distemper virus determined by the algorithm of Garnier, Osguthorpe and Robson. Turns are indicated in the figure; ▬▬▬ indicates a potential α-helical region and ∼ indicates a β-sheet prediction. Glycosylation sites are indicated by ↓. The secondary structure prediction is overprinted with antigenic indexes determined by the Jameson and Wolf algorithm.

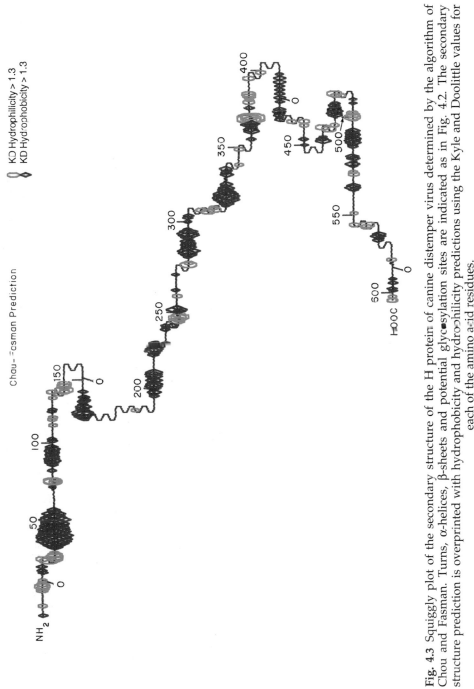

Chou-Fasman Prediction

◐ KD Hydrophilicity > 1.3
◇ KD Hydrophobicity > 1.3

Fig. 4.3 Squiggly plot of the secondary structure of the H protein of canine distemper virus determined by the algorithm of Chou and Fasman. Turns, α-helices, β-sheets and potential glycosylation sites are indicated as in Fig. 4.2. The secondary structure prediction is overprinted with hydrophobicity and hydrophilicity predictions using the Kyle and Doolittle values for each of the amino acid residues.

available to apply the physical techniques necessary for structural analysis and often only the primary sequence (derived from nucleic acid sequencing) is known. In this case, only predictions of the secondary structure can be made. The two most frequently used algorithms for this task have been developed by Chou and Fasman (1978) and by Garnier, Osguthorpe and Robson (1978). The former based their analysis on the potential of a given amino acid residue to form one of four conformational states, e.g. α-helix, β-sheet, random coil and reverse turn. Garnier and his colleagues modified the method, taking account of the effect that neighbouring amino acids have on the propensity of an amino acid to be in one of the conformational states. In a survey of 15 proteins of which the crystallographic structure had been determined, Chou and Fasman established the frequencies with which a given amino acid was found in any of the four conformational states. Predictions of the conformation of an unknown protein are then made by calculating the probabilities that a given stretch of amino acid residues has either of the four conformations. The conformation with the highest probability is then chosen as the predicted one. Unfortunately, these rules are somewhat biased by the crystallographic data set used. Thus the predictions work better for globular, soluble proteins than for membrane-associated or for homo- or heteropolymeric proteins or structural proteins from viruses and organelles. In a refinement of the prediction methodology Garnier and his co-workers (1978) took account of the effect that neighbouring amino acid residues up to 6–8 positions on either side have on the propensity of a given residue to be in an α-helix. This provides somewhat better predictions in a wider set of proteins with different shapes and properties.

Both programs provide data in the form of likely structures (see Fig. 4.1) at any position in the primary sequence or can be used to provide a 'squiggly' plot in which α-helix and β-sheet and turns are plotted in a two-dimensional graph (see Figs 4.2 and 4.3). In the latter two figures, squiggly plots of the same protein, the major antigenic protein (H) of canine distemper virus, are shown and the differences between the two predictions, one calculated by the Chou and Fasman rules and the other by the Garnier–Osguthorpe–Robson algorithm, indicate the fact that these plots must be interpreted with caution.

ANTIGENIC INDEX

It is recognised widely that the prediction of epitopes from the hydropathy or hydrophilicity indices, the surface probability or flexibility data is unreliable. Most researchers apply all the methods available and then make an informed guess at the sequence that most likely represents an epitope in the protein. A computer program has been developed by Jameson and Wolf (1988) to analyse this problem and to place a quantitative weighting on the parameters determined by the other programs. It defines an *antigenic index* on the basis of weighting the hydrophilicity (Hopp and Woods, 1981) value at a given residue, the flexibility and the logarithm of the surface probability and the secondary structure predictions by the Chou and Fasman (1978) and the Garnier *et al.* (1978) methods as follows. The program assigns a hydrophilicity H_i value of 2, 1, −1 or −2 depending on the values calculated by the Hopp and Woods program at any position being >0.5, 0.5 to 0, 0 to −0.4 or <−0.4, respectively. The log surface probability (S_i) and flexibility (F_i) are set at either 1 or 0 depending on the surface probability or flexibility being >1.0 or <1.0. Secondary structure predictions are weighted as follows: a strong turn predicted by Chou and Fasman or Garnier *et al.* gives CF_i and RG_i values of 2; to a residue in a weak turn or random coil a value of 1.0 is assigned and to any other structure a value of 0. The antigenic index is then calculated as:

$$A_i = 0.3(H_i) + 0.15(S_i) + 0.15(F_i) + 0.2(CF_i) + 0.2(RG_i)$$

All of these methods have been known to lead to wrong predictions, and the best strategy used by most researchers is to concentrate on areas of the protein sequence that give high values of hydrophilicity, antigenic index, surface probability and flexiblity and are predicted to be in turns of the secondary structure. Figure 4.1 demonstrates the outcome of this type of analysis for a particular sequence, in this case the attachment protein (H) of canine distemper virus (CDV). The output here is from the University of Wisconsin 'Genetics Computation Group's' program on peptide structure devised by John Devereux and co-workers (1984). The primary sequence of the H protein of CDV has been analysed by the various programs described above. Between amino acid residues 380 and 390 there is a peak in hydrophilicity (see also on the 'squiggly' plots in Figs 4.2 and 4.3), flexibility, surface probability and the antigenic index, and the sequence is predicted to be in an α-helix by both secondary structure prediction programs. It is thus considered to be a good candidate for a B-cell epitope. We also know that an alignment of all the paramyxovirus H proteins in this area shows no conserved residues, and even comparisons between the closely related morbilliviruses such as measles, CDV and rinderpest virus also show little conservation. Furthermore, we know from studies with a peptide of the H protein of measles virus representing this area that monospecific peptide antisera to this region react with the intact protein and that this area is on the surface of the molecule (see later, this chapter). In addition, monoclonal antibody escape mutants of measles virus have been mapped to this area and thus the prediction programs and the arguments about alignments and comparisons of related viruses suggest that one of the B-cell epitopes of the H protein of CDV would be located in this region. However, the plots in Fig. 4.1 indicate that this would have been only one of many areas predicted by the antigenic index program and additional information on peptide antisera, sequence diversity in different strains and monoclonal antibody escape mutants was thus useful in the delineation of this antigenic region of the H protein of CDV.

T-CELL EPITOPES

In Chapter 3 you will have seen that a T-cell epitope consists of a small oligopeptide fragment of a foreign antigen which has been proteolytically processed in *antigen-presenting cells* (APC), so that it can be presented to the T-cells after binding to a molecule of the major histocompatibility classes I or II (MHC in the mouse; HLA in human beings). This definition immediately emphasises that T-cell epitopes are actually defined by the major histocompatibility proteins and therefore a sequence which is recognised by T-cells in an animal of one histocompatibility type may not be recognised in another type. Nevertheless, predictive programs have been developed based on localised secondary structure predictions and the requirement for a peptide which is part of a T-cell epitope to be able to form an amphipathic helix, i.e. one with separate hydrophobic and hydrophilic surfaces. Other programs have been developed which take no account of secondary structure predictions but search the primary sequence for motifs, such as:

(Charged or Gly)-Φ-Φ-(polar or Gly)
or
(Charged or Gly)-Φ-Φ-(Φ- or Pro)-(polar or Gly)

where Φ is a hydrophobic amino acid residue. The existence of primary sequence patterns that are capable of predicting T-cell epitopes is surprising since they are restricted by MHC or HLA type as well as species, but, nevertheless, the search for these motifs has delineated T-cell epitopes in many proteins in several animal species. Now that the structure of some of the MHC and HLA determinants is known, it has become possible to refine the above-mentioned motifs into specific sub-patterns that would predict the ability of a particular primary sequence to interact with an MHC molecule and act as a T-cell epitope. By sequencing of random peptides bound to MHC molecules it has recently become possible to analyse rapidly the most likely residues in any particular position in the epitope. This knowledge should greatly enhance our ability to predict epitopes presented by particular MHC molecules.

COMPARATIVE NUCLEOTIDE SEQUENCE ANALYSIS

A final method which has been used, so far primarily for the identification of B-cell epitopes on microorganisms from which a large number of different strains or isolates are available, is the comparison of nucleotide sequences and deduced amino acid sequences of the proteins that are immunogenic. It has been recognised, for example, with picornaviruses such as poliovirus and foot-and-mouth disease virus that areas of variability in the sequence correspond to immunogenic epitopes. This reflects the observation that those parts of the amino acid sequences that most often change under immunological pressure will form part of the major epitopes in a particular molecule. In this way, for example, the major antigenic site on the VP1 of poliovirus type 3 was predicted to consist of amino acid residues 98–105 because of the sequence variation in this region. This method has been most successfully used in the case of viruses from which different serotypes and many variants were available, whereas for other viruses such as mumps and measles virus which are monotypic, i.e. where only one serotype is found, this approach has been unrewarding.

IDENTIFICATION OF EPITOPES

The availability of structural information about a particular antigen in the form of an X-ray crystallographic three-dimensional description is of great help in determining epitopes on a particular protein, and most of what we know about the positions of particular epitopes has been gained from determining the immunogenic regions of known model antigens for which a structure had been described. The major examples of relevance to the subject area of this book are the descriptions of the epitopes on the *haemagglutinin* and *neuraminidase* molecules of influenza virus and on poliovirus (see Chapter 6).

If such information is not available, different approaches have to be taken to define the epitopes on antigenic molecules. The first involves fragmentation of the antigen and analysis of the capacity of various fragments to bind serum or a monoclonal antibody. The second involves the isolation and sequence analysis of mutants of the organisms that have lost the particular epitopes, especially the isolation and characterisation of monoclonal antibody escape mutants. Thirdly, the development of peptide synthesis *pin technology* has allowed epitope scanning to be developed. Most of these techniques rely on the availability of monoclonal antibodies to a given antigen and in particular of such antibodies that react with linear, non-conformational epitopes.

FRAGMENTATION OF THE ANTIGEN

Delineation of epitopes can take place by analysis of the fragments of a protein that bind monoclonal antibodies. The fragmentation can be complete, as in the case of chemical cleavage of the antigen with cyanogen bromide. Chemical action on the methionine residues of a protein cleaves it into a number of fragments which can be fractionated by high-performance liquid chromatography (HPLC) or by sodium dodecyl sulphate polyacrylamide gel electrophoresis (SDS–PAGE) on gels. The fragments or a blot of the gel can then be analysed by assessing their ability to bind monoclonal antibodies or sera in *ELISA tests,* to be precipitated with specific antisera or monoclonal antibody or detected by *Western blotting techniques.* Fractions of a peptide antigen that bind the monoclonal antibody can then be further fragmented or directly sequenced by gas-phase sequencing in order to determine the position of the epitope. It is also possible to combine this approach with limited proteolysis methods described by Cleveland and his co-workers (1977). In this case the fragments derived from the antigen by treatment with a range of proteolytic enzymes are analysed by SDS–PAGE, and Western blots are analysed for monoclonal antibody binding capacity. These techniques are dependent on the availability of a large amount of antigen.

However, when cDNA clones that can express the proteins are available more rapid techniques based on genetic manipulation of the DNA and *in vivo* and *in vitro* expression of the proteins are applicable. For example, it is possible to make directed deletions of the cDNA clones in order to determine rapidly in which part of the expressed protein the linear epitope lies. It is further possible with modern nucleic acid techniques to make nested sets of deletions in such an expressed cDNA clone in order to determine which part of the total molecule binds the monoclonal antibody. Recently this idea has been modified by making fusion proteins (see Chapter 2) of random fragments of the antigen and selecting and sequencing clones that bind the monoclonal antibody. These techniques require the re-introduction of the altered cDNA clones into eukaryotic or prokaryotic organisms. The monoclonal antibody binding site on a particular protein can be determined even more rapidly, when a cDNA clone of the protein is coupled to bacteriophage promoters like those of phage T7 and T3. *In vitro* transcription of the cDNA clone into RNA can be followed by *in vitro* translation in the presence of radioactive precursors. The products can then be immunoprecipitated or Western blotted after SDS–PAGE. This can identify quickly which parts of the molecule bind the monoclonal antibody.

ANALYSIS OF MONOCLONAL ANTIBODY ESCAPE MUTANTS

Particularly with viruses, it is possible to exploit the relatively simple and rapid isolation of mutants when one wants to define the epitope to which neutralising monoclonal antibodies bind. Cultivation of the virus in the presence of such monoclonal antibodies allows the selection of escape mutants. Sequence analysis of the mutants then allows the identification of the areas of the amino acid sequence that are involved in binding the antibody used for selection. A further modification of this technique allows also the generation of escape mutants resistant to non-neutralising antibodies. By incubation of the cells in which viruses are being cultivated with complement it is possible to select mutants that escape binding the monoclonal antibody. This technique can also be used when the antibody for which one wants to establish the binding site is conformational. However, in this case the information obtained from the nucleotide sequence analysis only gives a very partial indication of the residues involved in the epitope. In such a situation sequence data can also identify those amino acid residues that are important in folding the protein chain into the conformation which gives rise to the epitope.

EPITOPE SCANNING TECHNIQUES

Solid-phase peptide synthesis techniques have been developed in the past decade. That allow the synthesis of a large number of small amounts of particular peptides on a solid support. With the original development of solid-phase peptide synthesis came the possibility to link the growing peptide chains to polystyrene pins embedded in a matrix so that one pin fits in the well of a conventional 96-well microtitre plate. This procedure is now called *pin technology*. The procedure allows the synthesis of a series of small overlapping peptides derived from the sequence of a protein. The small peptides attached to the pins may then be analysed for their ability to bind antibodies by the use of conventional immunological assays in microtitre plates. Those peptides containing the amino acid sequence of the monoclonal antibody binding site will bind antibody and a further delineation can then be made by synthesising a series of shorter peptides in this region of the sequence. This technique allows the rapid characterisation of linear epitopes in proteins from which the primary sequence is known, as indicated in the example given in Table 4.3.

Table 4.3 Example of an epitope scan: part of the CDV H protein sequence

Pin no.	Peptide sequence on the pin	Binding of mAb
A1	ALASSEKQQEEQKG	−
A2	LASSEKQQEEQKGC	−
A3	ASSEKQQEEQKGCL	+
A5	SSEKQQEEQKGCLE	+
A6	SEKQQEEQKGCLES	+
A7	EKQQEEQKGCLESA	++
A8	KQQEEQKGCLESAC	++
A9	QQEE**QKGCL**ESACQ	+++
A10	QEEQKGCLESACQR	++
A11	EEQKGCLESACQRK	+
A12	EQKGCLESACQRKT	+
B1	QKGCLESACQRKT Y	−
B2	KGCLESACQRKTYP	−
B3	GCLESACQRKTYPM	−
B4	CLESACQRKTYPM C	−
B5	LESACQRKTYPM CN	−

Part of the CDV H protein sequence also used in Figs 4.1, 4.2 and 4.3 is synthesised as a set of overlapping peptides linked to polystyrene pins. Binding of a monoclonal antibody (mAb) to the various peptides (pins) is quantified and the mAb binds only to those peptides which contain the linear epitope EQKGCL. A recent modification of this idea involves expressing all possible random hexapeptides in phage libraries and selecting and sequencing clones that bind monoclonal antibodies to determine their epitope.

A similar approach can also be used for the delineation of T-cell epitopes in a particular protein. However, the assays require the solubilisation of the peptide and binding to molecules of the major histocompatibility complex, and this thus necessitates removal of the peptides from the polystyrene pin. Recently, methods involving spacer arms that contain specific cleavable sequences have been developed to obtain the peptides in solution so that they can be used in *proliferation or chromium release assays* for the major T-cell activities.

SUMMARY

For the prediction of linear B-cell epitopes, a number of computer programs have been developed by analysis of the localisation and properties of amino acid residues in a set of proteins from which the three-dimensional structure has been determined by X-ray crystallography. Properties analysed are the hydrophobicity of residues, their probability to be on the surface of the molecule or their flexibility. Secondary structure predictions are made on the basis of the propensities of various amino acids to be in α-helix, β-sheet, random coil or β-turns. A composite program has been developed which calculates an antigenic index by weighting the values predicted by the other programs.

T-cell epitopes can be predicted on the basis of the amphipathicity of helices and on the basis of primary structure motifs. Epitopes can also be identified by studying sequence diversity in antigenic proteins. Epitopes can be localised in parts of the proteins by fragmentation of the antigen or by expression of partially deleted or truncated antigens generated by cloning technology. The binding of these fragments to monoclonal antibodies or their ability to induce T-cell proliferation can be assessed. Solid-phase peptide synthesis using pin technology can then be used to identify epitopes unambiguously.

SUGGESTED READING

Chou PY and Fasman GD (1978) Prediction of the secondary structure of proteins from their amino acid sequence. In: Meister A (ed.) *Advances in Enzymology*, pp. 45–148. New York: Wiley.

Cleveland DW, Fisher SG, Kirschner MW and Laemmli UK (1977) Peptide mapping by limited proteolysis in sodium dodecyl sulphate and analysis by gelelectrophoresis. *J. Biol. Chem.* **252**, 1102–1106.

Devereux J, Haeberli P and Smithies O (1984) A comprehensive set of sequence analysis programmes for the VAX. *Nucl. Acid Res.* **12**, 387–395.

Emini EA, Hughes JV, Perlow DS and Boger J (1985) Induction of hepatitis A virus-neutralising antibody by a virus-specific synthetic peptide. *Journal of Virology* **55**, 836–838.

Garnier J, Osguthorpe DJ and Robson B (1978) Analysis of the accuracy and implications of simple methods for predicting the secondary structure of globular proteins. *Journal of Molecular Biology* **120**, 97–120.

Hopp TP and Woods KR (1981) Prediction of the protein antigenic determinants from amino acid sequences. *Proceedings of the National Academy of Sciences USA* **78**, 3824–3828.

Jameson BA and Wolf H (1988) The antigenic index: A novel algorithm for predicting antigenic determinants. *CABIOS* **4**, 181–186.

Janin J, Wodak S, Levitt M and Maigret B (1978) Conformation of amino acid side-chains in proteins. *J. Mol. Biol.* **125**, 357–386.

Karplus PA and Schulz GE (1985) Prediction of chain flexibility in proteins. *Naturwissenschaften* **72**, 212–213.

Kyte J and Doolittle RF (1982) A simple method for displaying the hydropathic character of a protein. *Journal of Molecular Biology* **157**, 105–132.

Rothbard JB and Taylor WR (1988) A sequence pattern common to T cell epitopes. *EMBO Journal* **7**, 93–100.

5 Peptides as Vaccines

INTRODUCTION

The earliest vaccines to be developed, namely those produced against smallpox by Jenner in 1798, and chicken cholera, anthrax and rabies by Pasteur in 1880, 1881 and 1885 respectively, depended for their success on the multiplication of the weakened or attenuated organisms so that they evoked the protective immune responses without causing clinical disease. However, as long ago as the turn of the century it had been established that protection could also be obtained with the suitably inactivated organism or even a subunit of it. Heat-killed vaccines against typhoid fever, cholera and the plague had been prepared and the first of these had been used to immunise troops embarking for the Boer War in South Africa. Thus the principle had been established that non-replicating organisms could provide protection against the diseases they caused.

But as mentioned in Chapter 1, of greater significance was Behring's discovery that toxins secreted from the bacteria causing tetanus and diphtheria could be used to produce antitoxin sera that passively protected against these diseases, which earned him the first Nobel Prize in Physiology or Medicine in 1901. Some years later the same toxins, detoxified with formaldehyde, were used in man for active immunisation. Thus it was established that the entire microorganism was not necessary to afford protection.

Until about 30 years ago little had been done to extend these observations, probably because of the lack of knowledge of the detailed composition and structure of the infecting organisms, with some notable exceptions such as tobacco mosaic virus and MS2 bacteriophage. However, since the 1950s, with the development of methods for the growth of viruses in large amounts outside the animal body and the means to label them with radioactive precursors, together with improved methods to purify and analyse virus particles and their sub-components, basic structural information began to accumulate rapidly. Moreover, methods to dissect viruses into biologically active subunits were also developed. Of particular importance in the context of this chapter was the observation that protective immunity could be achieved, at least in experimental animals, by the inoculation of the surface projections of several lipid-containing viruses, including those causing influenza, measles, rabies and vesicular stomatitis (see review by Brown, 1984). At about the same time methods were being developed to analyse proteins. These methods, and particularly polyacrylamide gel electrophoresis

(PAGE), have allowed us to identify rapidly the protein or proteins of a virus which elicit the protective immune response.

We will now examine the current success of the synthetic immunogen approach and will illustrate the way that the principles of epitope prediction and identification outlined in the previous chapter have been utilised in specific situations.

SYNTHETIC IMMUNOGENS

As the next step in this process of reductionism, it was shown by Anderer in 1963 that small fragments of the protein of tobacco mosaic virus, obtained by cleavage enzymes, would inhibit the reaction between the virus and its antibody and could also elicit antibody which neutralised the infectivity of the virus. Tobacco mosaic virus is rod-shaped, measuring 300×18 nm, and consists of one molecule of positive-sense RNA, molecular weight 2×10^6, and 2200 copies of a single protein of molecular weight 18×10^3, consisting of 158 amino acids. The amino acid sequence of the protein had been determined by amino acid sequencing methods only in 1960, and it was possible to synthesise the fragment by the then laborious and difficult methods of peptide chemistry. Of considerable importance was the fact that the short synthetic peptides corresponding to the C-terminus, coupled to bovine serum albumin, would elicit the formation of antibodies which not only precipitated the virus but also neutralised its infectivity. This work was a major step in our understanding of vaccination because it provided the first example of a synthetic immunogen and established the principle that short peptides had potential as synthetic vaccines.

Anderer's work on tobacco mosaic virus was followed by Sela and his colleagues, using MS2 coliphage as a model, providing further evidence that fragments of a viral protein would evoke antibodies which reacted with the intact protein on the virus particle. *MS2 coliphage* is a 23 nm diameter icosahedral particle consisting of one copy of a single-stranded RNA molecule, molecular weight 1.2×10^6, 180 copies of a coat protein consisting of 129 amino acids and a single copy of protein A, molecular weight $35-44 \times 10^3$. Treatment of the coat protein with cyanogen bromide, which cleaves at methionine residues, yielded three fragments. The fragment comprising residues 89–108 strongly inhibited the reaction between the virus and its antibody. Moreover, a synthetic peptide corresponding to this fragment, coupled to poly-DL-alanyl-poly(DL-lysine), induced antibodies which reacted with the virus particle. These experiments with tobacco mosaic virus and MS2 phage pointed the way to the possibility of synthetic peptide vaccines.

The main reason for the delay in exploiting this breakthrough quickly was the lack of information on the amino acid sequences of the immunogenic proteins of other viruses and pathogens. Apart from those for tobacco mosaic virus and MS2 bacteriophage, no amino acid sequences for viral proteins were available until the nucleic acid sequencing methods of Maxam and Gilbert and Sanger and his colleagues became available in 1977 (see Chapter 2). These major breakthroughs in molecular biology revolutionised our approaches to vaccine development. From 1977 onwards, sequences for a multitude of proteins have been derived from the corresponding nucleic acid sequences. At the same time, studies on the replication of viruses had identified the genes coding for the individual proteins. This information, together with the major steps that had been made in manipulating DNA fragments so that they could be expressed in a variety of organisms, provided rich new sources of proteins. This advance was particularly valuable in those instances where the protein or infectious agent could not be produced in the laboratory in the amounts required for vaccine production, such as the agents causing hepatitis B and malaria.

By the early 1980s, considerable information on the molecular biology of foot-and-mouth disease virus had become available, and Anderer's approach was used by Strohmaier and his colleagues in Tübingen. Foot-and-mouth disease virus consists of one molecule of single-stranded RNA, molecular weight 2.6×10^6, and 60 copies of each of four proteins with molecular weight 24×10^3 for VP1, VP2 and VP3 and 10×10^3 for VP4. Inactivated virus particles are highly immunogenic, only 10 µg in a *single* inoculation being required to fully protect a cow against a severe challenge infection. The major immunogenic site appears to be located on VP1 because cleavage of this *in situ* with proteolytic enzymes such as trypsin or chymotrypsin leads to a considerable loss of immunogenic activity with many isolates of the virus. Strohmaier's group cleaved VP1 by two methods to obtain biologically active fragments: firstly, *in situ* with various proteolytic enzymes; and secondly, with cyanogen bromide. From an analysis of the immunogenicity of the separate fragments, they concluded that the sequences 146–154 and 200–213 contained active sites.

However, these were early days in novel approaches to vaccination and the important issue of the immunogenic activity of the fragments compared with that of the intact viruses was not studied by these groups of workers. Not only is this important if the peptides were to be used commercially, but it is also basic to our understanding of the configuration necessary to evoke the relevant immune response. This problem will be considered below.

SOLVENT-ACCESSIBLE REGIONS AND SECONDARY STRUCTURE

As mentioned in Chapter 4, the main guideline to the location of immunogenic sequences on protein molecules is that the sites will be on the surface and therefore likely to be hydrophilic. Various procedures have been developed to assist with the identification of epitope sites and these have been applied with limited success to various virus proteins. With viruses, however, there is the additional consideration that the interaction of the immunogenic protein with the other proteins of the particle and with the nucleic acid will impose conformational constraints that analysis of the individual protein will not reveal. Not surprisingly therefore, several of the maxima predicted by Hopp and Woods' plots for tobacco mosaic virus protein and for the VP1 of foot-and-mouth disease virus did not correspond to immunogenic regions. However, when the correlation between antigenicity and hydrophilicity was analysed by the Chou–Fasman helix predictions and the Garnier B-strand prediction, agreement was substantial, but with respect to only the highest peaks. Consequently it seems preferable to consider only the highest peaks in hydrophilicity plots.

It is also known that flexible regions of proteins are more immunogenic than other regions. This flexibility may account for the high level of antibody elicited by foot-and-mouth disease virus vaccines that is directed towards the 141–160 region of VP1, which is now known from its three-dimensional structure to be exposed and highly flexible. Moreover, peptides corresponding to this sequence are highly immunogenic, a few micrograms being sufficient to elicit protective levels of neutralising antibody in experimental animals. In fact, the ability of short peptides to react with antibodies directed to mobile regions of the protein probably reflects the steric complementarity which exists when they possess sufficient mobility to adapt to a pre-existing paratope.

It has also been suggested that the main reason why certain segments of a protein are antigenic is because of their pronounced surface exposure. Calculations show a protrusion index for each amino acid that reflects the degree to which it protrudes from the surface of a number of proteins whose tertiary structure are known. The regions which protruded were found to correlate with the positions of continuous epitopes.

In many proteins the N- and C-termini are located at the surface of the molecule. Because of their position, these regions are less constrained than internal segments and have a high relative flexibility. This probably accounts for the presence of continuous epitopes at the termini of many proteins.

ANTIGENIC AND SEQUENCE VARIABILITY

In families of homologous proteins, high sequence variability often corresponds to the location of epitopes. Moreover, regions of a protein which can change in conformation without affecting the folding of the molecule are likely to be on the surface. Natural selection also favours those amino acid substitutions that do not perturb the overall tertiary structure of the proteins, that is, those that occur in highly accessible mobile regions.

The value of the method for epitope prediction is well illustrated by the example of foot-and-mouth disease virus. The virus occurs as seven serotypes, with a mutiplicity of subtypes within serotypes. Comparison of the sequences of the immunogenic protein VP1 of several isolates showed that considerable sequence variation occurs at positions 41–60, 134–160 and 195–204. The first region is somewhat hydrophobic although the other two are hydrophilic. Peptides to the 134–160 and 195–204 regions elicited high levels of antipeptide antibody but only 134–160 evoked a high level of neutralising antibody. More recent X-ray crystallographic studies (Acharya *et al.*, 1989) revealed that both these sequences are on the surface of the virus particle, with the 134–160 region constituting a highly exposed and flexible loop region, thus meeting the predicted requirements for a continuous epitope.

An extension of this method has been described in which antigenic variants were isolated by growing poliovirus or influenza virus in the presence of neutralising monoclonal antibodies. Comparison of the sequences of the parent and the escape mutant viruses identified the sites involved in neutralisation. However, this may be an oversimplified approach because it has been found with foot-and-mouth disease virus, for example, that internal substitutions in the 41–60 region of VP1 can influence the reactivity of the 134–160 surface loop region. Other examples have also been described in which the reactivity of epitopes has been altered by substitutions elsewhere in the protein.

ANTIGEN–ANTIBODY COMPLEXES

Much information could undoubtedly be obtained by the study of the crystal structure of antigen–antibody complexes. There are a few examples of such studies, notably with lysozyme and with the *neuraminidase* of influenza virus, which represent major advances in our understanding of antigen–antibody interaction. Moreover, site-directed mutagenesis of both antigen and antibody should lead to detailed information on the contribution of individual amino acids to their interaction. Clearly the high level of sophistication necessary for these studies will mean that the number of antigens which can be examined in this way will be limited, at least in the immediate future. However, the rapid advances made during the past decade in methods for solving protein structures may mean that this view is unduly pessimistic if the present rate of advance is maintained.

PRESENTATION OF PEPTIDES TO THE HOST

It was long considered that it would be necessary to link peptides to a carrier protein such as keyhole limpet haemocyanin or tetanus toxoid if they were to function as immunogens. There is now ample evidence that peptides alone can be immunogenic provided that they include a T-cell epitope appropriate for the recipient species. Nevertheless most peptides have been linked to a carrier protein before presentation to the recipient. The linkers most frequently used are: (a) glutaraldehyde; (b) carbodiimides; (c) bisdiazobenzidine; and (d) maleimidobenzoyl *N*-hydroxysuccinimide ester.

This subject is reviewed comprehensively by van Regenmortel *et al.* (1988) in an excellent publication.

On theoretical grounds it would seem logical to ensure that the amino acid involved in attachment should occur only once in the peptide, preferably at a terminus. Thus glutaraldehyde, which forms links between NH_2 groups, should be avoided when lysine residues occupy a central position in the peptide. Similarly, carbodiimides, which link —COOH to —NH_2 groups, should not be used when aspartic and glutamic acid residues are present in the middle of the peptide. Bis-diazobenzidine, which reacts with tyrosine residues, and maleimidobenzoyl *N*-hydroxysuccinimide ester, which reacts with cysteine residues, should not be used when these amino acids are centrally placed. In fact, it is logical to include a residue suitable for attachment at one of the termini of the peptide, even though it does not form part of the natural sequence. Cysteine and tyrosine residues in particular have been used for this purpose.

It was mentioned above that attachment to a carrier protein was not a necessary requirement for a peptide to be immunogenic. What seems to be necessary, however, is the need to have multiple copies of the peptide in a single molecule. Thus, the peptide corresponding to residues 141–160 of VP1 of foot-and-mouth disease virus is not immunogenic but it is active when (a) polymerised with glutaraldehyde, (b) dimerised by incorporating a cysteine residue at the C-terminus, (c) polymerised by oxidation of cysteine residues added at each end of the molecule, or (d) when synthesised as a tetramer or octamer on a poly-lysine backbone.

Linking of a peptide to a carrier protein can also be achieved by ligating the genes coding for them and expressing the hybrid gene in a suitable expression system. One example of this approach which proved to be valuable was the expression of the 141–160 sequence of VP1 of foot-and-mouth disease virus attached to the N-terminus of hepatitis B virus core protein. This system took advantage of the fact that the core protein self-assembles into 27 nm particles even when foreign amino acids are attached to either terminus. Such a construction thus ensures that multiple copies of the added antigen are presented on a particle. In this particular example in which the foot-and-mouth disease virus sequence is attached to the N-terminus, the neutralising antibody response was greatly enhanced. Whereas about 100µg of the peptide, attached via an added cysteine to keyhole limpet haemocyanin, were required to evoke a protective level of neutralising antibody in guinea pigs, only 0.2µg was required when it was presented on the hepatitis B virus core.

Initially, many workers dismissed peptides as potential vaccines because the immune response they induced was low compared with that evoked by the protein or virus particle. However, it is becoming increasingly apparent that by presenting the peptide in a conformation similar to that which it has in the native protein much better responses are obtained. Antibodies recognise conformations and not the sequences which constitute them. For example, antisera prepared against fragments of ribonuclease react well with the fragments but poorly with the enzyme itself. Conversely, antibodies against the native protein react weakly with the fragments. This can be explained by assuming that the fragments exist in a range of conformations, only a small proportion of which may resemble the conformation of the corresponding region on the native protein. In contrast, we have found that with the antibodies elicited by the 141–160 peptide of VP1 of foot-and-mouth disease virus, the virus particle absorbed 30% of the antipeptide activity. This result suggests that the G–H loop region of the virus, which is known to be flexible as well as immunodominant, is mimicked well by the peptide and may account for its ability to elicit high levels of neutralising antibody.

Further evidence that conformation is important was shown by the enhanced immunogenicity of a predicted loop region of hepatitis B virus surface antigen corresponding to amino acids 117–137 following the introduction of a disulphide bond between the cysteine residues at positions 125 and 137. In a more sophisticated study Muller et al. (1990) showed that by imposing on residues 139–147 of the antigenic site A of influenza haemagglutinin, a constrained loop structure which was essentially identical to its structure on the protein itself, an immune response could be obtained in mice which protected them against lethal infection. Studies on the conformation of antigenic sequences within a protein molecule can thus be very rewarding. As more structural data become available it should be increasingly possible to carry out experiments similar to those of Muller and his colleagues.

GENETIC RESTRICTION

As mentioned above, it had been expected that peptides would behave like haptens and would only be immunogenic if attached to a carrier protein. However, it has become clear that peptides alone are highly immunogenic provided they contain sites which stimulate antibody production. That is, they must contain T-helper cell epitopes in addition to the specific antibody recognition sites or B-cell epitopes (see Chapter 3). The T-cell epitopes must be able to bind class II major histocompatibility complex (MHC) molecules on the surface of the antigen-presenting cells of the host and the B-cells (see Chapter 3). They must subsequently interact with the T-cell receptor so that they induce the B-cells to proliferate.

Because T-cells recognize 'processed' fragments of protein antigens, the problem of conformation is probably avoided. However, there are other constraints imposed by the T-cells because there is the problem of dual recognition of the 'processed' antigen plus the MHC molecules. The T-cell response appears to be focused on a limited number of determinants. The number of potential T-cell sites is probably not the limiting factor but the sites selected by the individual MHC haplotype. The basic problem is to identify T-cell epitopes that are suitable for a particular species. With animals whose genetic background is well defined this is not too large a task. However, when there has been extensive cross-breeding, as in most human populations, the problem is greater. In one experimental system using mice of the H-2d haplotype, it was found that their failure to respond to the 141–160 peptide of foot-and-mouth disease virus could be overcome by covalently linking to it a sequence from sperm whale myoglobin or ovalbumin. Similar experiments with peptides from the malaria circumsporozoite, rotavirus and hepatitis B virus have demonstrated the effectiveness of this approach. Hence, although the problem of species-specific immunogenetic restriction is considerable there is good evidence that the task is not insurmountable.

SUMMARY

The practical and theoretical advantages of peptide vaccines, compared with the vaccines in current use, would be enormous. Not only would the products be readily produced and indefinitely stable but they would avoid the inoculation of those parts of a protein or virus which bear no relevance to immunity. Clearly there are several problems to be solved. For example, the conformation of the B-cell epitope is extremely important. Overcoming genetic restriction is probably an even more challenging problem because studies on the structural basis for the interaction of T-cell epitopes with the MHC molecules are in their infancy. Understanding the time scale of protection and the consequences of subsequent infection remain to be determined. However, our increasing knowledge of the molecular structure of pathogens and in particular of the structure and conformation of their antigens and the way in which the immune system responds to them provides us with a new and rational approach to vaccine development and design that was not available to the discoverers of vaccination.

SUGGESTED READING

Acharya R, Fry E, Stuart D, Fox G, Rowlands DJ and Brown F (1989) The three-dimensional structure of foot-and-mouth disease virus at 2.9 A resolution. *Nature* **337**, 709–716.

Bittle JL, Houghten RA, Alexander H, Shinnick TM, Sutcliffe JG, Lerner RA, Rowlands DJ and Brown F (1982) Protection against foot-and-mouth disease by immunisation with a chemically synthesised peptide predicted from the viral nucleotide sequence. *Nature* **298**, 30–33.

Brown F (1984) Synthetic viral vaccines. *Annual Review of Microbiology* **38**, 221–235.

Muller S, Plaue S, Samama JP, Valette M, Briand JP and van Regenmortel MHV (1990) Antigenic properties and protective capacity of a cyclic peptide corresponding to site A of influenza virus haemagglutinin. *Vaccine* **8**, 308–314.

Van Regenmortel MHV, Briand JP, Muller S and Plaue S (1988) Synthetic polypeptides as antigens. In: Burdon RH and van Knippenberg PH (eds) *Laboratory Techniques in Biochemistry and Molecular Biology*. New York: Elsevier.

6 Vaccines Against Virus Diseases

INTRODUCTION

For the purpose of this book it is most instructive to consider the relationship between the knowledge that has been obtained about the surface structure of viruses and their antigenicity. This should give us an insight into the immunogenic regions of viral surfaces and allow the possible development of viral subunit vaccines for specific applications (for example, such as those in immunocompromised hosts) and the possible determination of viral structures that should be inserted in other vectors in order to elicit an appropriate immune response. Surface structures will be described in detail for some viruses, representing non-enveloped and enveloped viruses. How viruses can evade the immune system will also be described. First we describe some current used viral vaccines.

CURRENT VIRAL VACCINES

Vaccines against virus diseases are among the most successful immunoprophylactic agents and their application has led to the control of many diseases at least in those countries that have been able to afford and organise effective immunisation programmes. The success of virus vaccines is illustrated in Fig. 6.1, which shows the effect of vaccination with measles vaccine in the USA on the annual number of cases reported. This illustrates clearly the ability of a vaccination programme to suppress the incidence of a viral disease.

Viral vaccines are either based on live-attenuated virus strains which are able to infect the patients without leading to clinical manifestations or they are based on inactivated viruses or subunits of viruses. Live-attenuated viral vaccines are among the most successful and these can provide life-long protection for the vaccinee. Although in some cases there are side-effects which may be severe in a small proportion of the vaccinees (perhaps one in a million doses) in most cases they are absent or at least so slight that the balance between the benefits of the vaccination outweigh the associated clinical symptoms. Live-attenuated forms of the viruses have the advantage that they often elicit immune reactions involving both arms of the immune system and therefore provide better protection. Ideally they contain a large number of T- and B-cell epitopes that give rise to large populations of memory cells and maintain high levels of neutralising antibody to

54

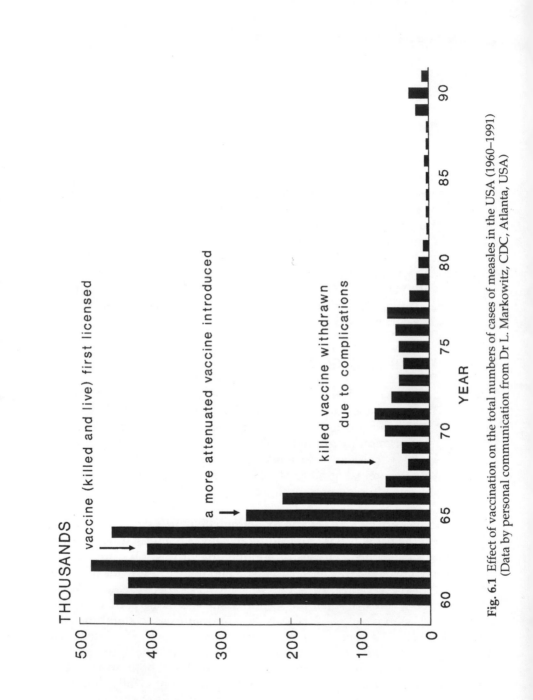

Fig. 6.1 Effect of vaccination on the total numbers of cases of measles in the USA (1960–1991) (Data by personal communication from Dr L. Markowitz, CDC, Atlanta, USA)

reduce the immediate effect of post-vaccination exposure to a virus. The fact that live-attenuated virus vaccines probably contain most or all of the T-cell epitopes also present in the wild virus strains and the fact that they can infect the same types of antigen-presenting cells is probably the reason for the better response to these vaccines than to inactivated viral preparations. Their major disadvantage is that there is a danger of reversion of the virus strains to more reactive and virulent forms. A clearer understanding of the differences at the molecular level between wild type and attenuated strains may indicate the likelihood of these events. These also lead to a requirement for extensive testing of batches of viral vaccines, often involving expensive and cumbersome animal tests. For example, in the case of the poliovirus vaccine a neurovirulence test in monkeys is required for all batches of vaccine. It is also sometimes difficult to correlate the level of protection that a vaccine must induce with the level of attenuation of the virus strain used. For example, in the case of infectious bronchitis of chickens, the first vaccination has to take place with a very high-passage and very attenuated virus before immune protection can be obtained using a lower-passage, less attenuated strain. Final protection in some specific animals then requires further inoculation with inactivated virus. In this case the protection clearly has to be built up slowly and by repeated inoculations with different virus preparations.

Table 6.1 Current viral vaccines in human and veterinary medicine

Type of vaccine	Medical use	Veterinary use
Live-attenuated	Vaccinia	Marek's disease
	Varicella zoster	Pseudorabies
	Adeno	Egg drop syndrome
		Feline inf. enteritis
	Measles	Rinderpest
	Mumps	Canine distemper
	Polio	Rabies
	Dengue	Newcastle disease
	Rubella	Bursal disease
		Bovine parainfluenza
	Respiratory syncytial virus	Bovine respiratory syncytial virus
Inactivated virus	Polio	Foot-and-mouth disease
	Influenza	Infect. bronchitis
	Rabies	Porcine parvovirus
		Pseudorabies
Subunit vaccine	Hepatitis B	
	Influenza	
Recombinant virus	–	Rabies
		Rinderpest
		Pseudorabies

Inactivated or subunit viral vaccines are also being developed or are in use (see Table 6.1). Inactivated virus vaccines are used primarily for those viruses which are easily and reliably inactivated. In particular the ease of inactivation of the nucleic acid is important in this respect and consequently viruses with an RNA genome are easier to inactivate than DNA viruses. Virus inactivation, however, is prone to failure and incidents with improperly inactivated poliovirus and foot-and mouth disease virus (FMDV) vaccines have highlighted this problem. Another problem with the preparation of such viral vaccines is that large amounts of pathogenic viral material are generated and thus high-security production plants are required to protect the workers and the environment from accidental exposure to the agents involved.

One alternative is the development of subunit vaccines based on specific viral proteins or parts of proteins or even small peptides. However, a disadvantage of subunit vaccines is that they may not contain a large enough number of T-cell epitopes to elicit immune responses in all members of the host population. Especially, when only one viral surface protein is capable of eliciting protective immune responses, viral subunit vaccines can be developed. Subunit vaccines are particularly useful in cases where attenuation has not been successful. This may be the result, for example, of the lack of required virus replication systems, or the danger of contamination of preparations with infectious viral nucleic acid or in the case of retroviruses because of fears of integration and mutation of the viruses.

Table 6.1 lists the current viral vaccines used in medicine and in the veterinary field. In general the primary approach to vaccination is the development of an attenuated strain of the virus, and live-attenuated vaccines are under trial or development for a number of viruses such as cytomegalovirus, human respiratory syncytial, dengue, influenza, hepatitis A and Japanese encephalitis viruses. Recombinant vaccines based on vaccinia and other viral vectors are currently under study for a number of veterinary and human viral vaccines (see Chapter 9).

VIRAL SURFACE STRUCTURES

For the development and design of subunit vaccines or vaccines for specific applications, knowledge about the immunogenic regions of viral antigens is essential. For many viral vaccines, surface antigens of the virus are among the most important to elicit neutralising antibodies and other appropriate humoral immune responses, although cell-mediated immunity is often associated with internal proteins. In this section we describe in detail the surface structures of picornaviruses and influenza viruses as examples of non-enveloped and enveloped viruses, respectively.

NON-ENVELOPED VIRUSES

Quite a number of animal virus families fall into this category, namely the Picornaviridae, Caliciviridae, Reoviridae, Parvoviridae, Papovaviridae, Reoviridae, Birnaviridae and the Adenoviridae. To date, most of the high-resolution X-ray crystallographic structural studies have been done with the picornaviruses, with examples of each genus having been analysed, and this discussion will be confined to this group.

The picornaviruses are a family of small animal viruses measuring between 25 and 30 nm in diameter. They were initially divided into four genera on the basis of physiochemical properties. The enterovirus genus contains the polioviruses, coxsackieviruses and the echoviruses, along with various enteroviruses of animals. Originally hepatitis A virus was included in this genus. However, sequencing studies have indicated that it is quite distinct from other members of this group and it is now suggested that it be placed into a fifth, separate genus. Some of the enteroviruses have the capability of causing severe medical and economic problems. Indeed it is only within the past 40 years that vaccination against poliomyelitis has almost completely eradicated this disease from the Western world. However, the ailment still remains a major hazard in many Third World areas, although it has been targeted for eradication by the World Health Organisation. A second genus, the rhinoviruses, contains approximately 200 serotypes of the common cold virus. Because of their diversity and widespread occurrence, these viruses probably cause more manpower-lost days in industry than any other type of virus, thus resulting in extensive economic loss. The cardioviruses comprise a family of viruses which normally only infect mice and therefore will not be considered in any further detail. The fourth genus, the aphthoviruses, comprises the foot-and-mouth disease viruses (FMDVs) which cause a severe disease in cattle. There are seven distinct serotypes of the virus which are endemic in various parts of the world.

Most picornaviruses (but not all) grow relatively well in tissue culture cells and can be purified easily. These properties have allowed them to be extensively studied at the structural, biological and molecular levels. Such studies have in part been motivated by the desire to get more reliable, cheap, safe and stable vaccines suitable for use in poorer countries of the world. Thus considerable effort has been devoted to determining the antigenic regions of the major disease-causing viruses and to relating these to the overall structure of the virus particle. The results of such efforts are described briefly below.

Mature picornavirus particles are comprised of a single-stranded RNA genome (7.5–8 kb) surrounded by a protein coat consisting of 60 copies of four polypeptide chains. These structural polypeptides are termed viral proteins (VP) 1, 2, 3 and 4. The first three are of approximately 25 000 molecular weight whereas VP4 is about 10 000 molecular weight. The virus capsid (protein coat) is composed of 60 subunits containing one copy of each of the viral proteins. The subunits are arranged with icosahedral symmetry, i.e. the capsid has 12, fivefold axes, 20 threefold axes and 30 twofold axes of rotational symmetry (Fig. 6.2). The fact that the picornavirus capsid possesses a regular icosahedral symmetry has facilitated the crystallisation of a number of them and as a result the three-dimensional structure of various virus representatives of four genera have been determined at high resolution. These include poliovirus (PV) type 1, human rhinovirus (HRV) 14, memgovirus and FMDV. The results have revealed a considerable structural similarity between picornaviruses and have given an insight into the structural basis of the antigenicity of these viruses. In each case the capsid is a spherical protein shell in which the proteins are situated at a radius of between approximately 100 and 150 Å from the centre. The orientation of the three principal structural proteins within the capsid are similar in each case. The VP1 proteins are clustered around each fivefold axis, whereas VP2 and VP3 alternate around each threefold axis (Fig. 6.2). In addition, all of the proteins have the same basic shape. They are wedged-shaped molecules with a core consisting of an eight-stranded antiparallel β-barrel which has

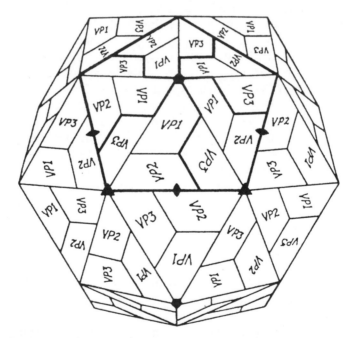

Fig. 6.2 Diagrammatic representation of the arrangement of the three major structural proteins in the icosahedral picornavirus capsid. Five copies of VP1 are situated around each fivefold axis of symmetry and three copies of VP1 and VP3 alternate around each sixfold axis of symmetry. Reprinted with permission from *Nature* **317**, 145–156. Copyright 1985 Macmillan Magazines Limited

two flanking helices. The eight strands which compose the front and back surfaces of the wedge are designated A–H. Each protein has different terminal extensions and internal insertions. The positions of such insertions are located in corresponding positions when equivalent proteins of different viruses are compared.

The solving of the structure of these viruses at high resolution would not have been possible without a knowledge of the amino acid sequence of the capsid proteins. Recent advances in gene cloning and nucleic acid sequencing techniques have permitted the elucidation of the complete sequence of the genomes of many viruses in this family and from these it has been possible to predict the amino acid sequences of the virus-encoded proteins. Sequence comparisons between viruses have indicated that the picornavirus structural proteins are the most diverse of the virus-encoded polypeptides. However, they do have regions of homology, possibly suggesting that they have all been derived from a common ancestor. These conserved regions tend to form the core parts of the proteins.

A knowledge of the sequence of the viral structural proteins has been essential for the determination of their antigenic structure. Two different strategies that have been employed for the elucidation of neutralising epitopes have confirmed the localisation of the antigenic sites on loops on the surface of the viruses. When the structural protein sequences of serotypes of the same virus are compared, conserved regions and variable regions are observed. Because the viruses differ antigenically, it is possible that at least some of these variable regions represent neutralising epitopes, differing in each virus serotype. To investigate this possibility various research groups have synthesised peptides corresponding to these regions and raised antisera against these. The ability of these sera to neutralise the parental virus have indicated the position of such sites. With some viruses the results of such experiments have been remarkably successful. For example, studies with FMDV have indicated the presence of two important epitopes in VP1 (residues 140–160 and 200–213). The amino acid sequences in these regions are very variable between strains. Similar work with a bovine enterovirus has indicated that important neutralising epitopes are situated on both VP2 and VP3. The elucidation of neutralising epitopes by this method is only possible if such sites are formed by amino acids occurring consecutively on any of the structural proteins; however, in many instances contributions to antigenic sites are made by residues from distal regions of the same protein or indeed by contributions from different proteins which are brought close together in the mature virus particle when the various proteins fold correctly.

An alternative approach, using neutralising monoclonal antibodies, has been used to investigate these sites. Picornaviruses are RNA viruses and are therefore susceptible to a higher rate of mutation than DNA viruses since RNA polymerases do not possess a proof-reading mechanism. If sufficient virus is grown in the presence of a neutralising monoclonal antibody then variants with mutations at the particular antigenic site recognised by the antibody will be the only viruses that will escape neutralisation. Sequence analysis of such viruses, termed *monoclonal antibody escape mutants*, define the residues contributing to that epitope. With a combination of both techniques the antigenic structures of a number of picornaviruses have been established. Generally there seem to be only four or five principal neutralising epitopes on each virus. The polioviruses have four, termed sites 1 to 4. However, because the capsid is built up from 60 subunits there are 60 copies of each epitope on each mature virus particle. The poliovirus sites differ in relative immunodominance between the three serotypes (PV1, 2 and 3). Their positions on the three structural proteins is given in Table 6.2, along with those of the four neutralising epitopes which occur on human rhinovirus (HRV-14). In the latter virus these have been termed *neutralisation immunogens* (NIm). A striking similarity exists in the antigenic structure of these two viruses. Site 1 in PV2 and PV3 is analogous to NIm-IA on HRV-14; site 2 of PV1 and PV3 is analogous to NIm-II; and site 4 of PV1 and PV3 is analogous to NIm-III. With FMDV, the epitopes detected on VP1 using peptide antisera have already been mentioned. The major immunodominant site occurs on VPI at amino acids 140–160. Another site is analogous to site 4 in PV. Further work with neutralising monoclonal antibodies have defined two additional epitopes on one strain of FMDV which have contributions from VP2 and VP3 residues, respectively. The former is analogous to site 3 on PV and NIm-III on HRV-14. However, there are variations between serotypes.

Table 6.2 Antigenic sites of poliovirus and HRV-14. The structural protein and the amino acid positions are given for each site for both viruses. It should be noted that there are differences between the three poliovirus serotypes (see text)

	Poliovirus	HRV-14	
Site 1	VPI 89–100, 140, 165, 255	NIm-IA NIm-IB	VP1 91–95 VP1 83-85,138,139
Site 2	VP2 160–170; VP1 220; C-terminus of VP2	NIm-II	VP2 158–162
Site 3	VP3 60–70; VP1 280–290		
Site 4	VP3 77–80; VP2 72	NIm-III	VP3 72–75, 78

As already stated, the major immunogenic sites of the picornaviruses have been shown to be localised on surface loops. For example, site 1 of PV and NIm-IA of HRV-14 both occur on the loop connecting β-strand B and C. The immunodominant region of FMDV also occurs as a surface loop which, because of disorder in the electron density maps obtained, as yet cannot be assigned definite structure. PV1 and HRV-14 both possess a surface depression called the canyon. It has been proposed that this is the site for cell attachment. The amino acid residues at the base of this site are highly conserved between virus strains and it is thought that the depression is too small to allow antibody access. Thus this region is shielded from immune surveillance, reducing the risk of mutations at this site. FMDV does not possess such a canyon; however, part of the cell attachment site constituting the residues Arg-Gly-Asp (RGD) is located in the principal neutralising epitope region (amino acids 140–160 of VP1). The RGD sequence is conserved in all but one FMDV, yet the rest of the region varies considerably, probably because of pressure to evade the immune response. Why then does the RGD sequence remain invariant? It has been proposed that it is maintained because it is camouflaged by the areas of high variability that occur around it. Another possibility is that the mutations at this site are lethal to the virus because the virus would then not be able to attach to its receptor; therefore only viruses containing the RGD sequence can survive and thus they are the only ones maintained in nature.

Thus it can be seen that considerable advances have been made in our understanding of the molecular basis of the antigenic structures of picornaviruses. How such knowledge is being applied to the development of novel vaccines is described in Chapter 9.

ENVELOPED VIRUSES

With the exception of influenza virus none of the surface structures of enveloped viruses have been described in the same amount of detail as the picornaviruses (see above). Thus the immunogenicity of many of the viral proteins presumed to be involved in eliciting the immune response required for successful vaccination cannot be assigned to specific molecular structures.

The structure of the two glycoproteins, the haemagglutinin and neuraminidase that form the outer coat of influenza virus type A have been known for almost a decade, and this knowledge has been very instructive in our understanding of the relationship between immunogenicity and three-dimensional structure of viral proteins. Influenza virus displays a phenomenon called antigenic drift, which results in variation of the coat proteins of various virus isolates. An indication that this process is driven by immunological pressure and not by random mutation is derived from the observed frequency of silent and non-silent mutations in natural isolates. In HA1 the rate of nucleotide exchange in expressed positions is 0.8% per annum while that in non-expressed positions is only 0.3%. In almost all comparisons of viral proteins the rate of silent mutation is much greater than that of expressed ones, and the inversion of this ratio is taken as an indication of immunological pressure. *Antigenic shift* is different from *antigenic drift,* since the latter involves the exchange of an entire fragment of the genome encoding one of the two glycoproteins with that of another virus by reassortment.

(a)

3 Leu-Phe
9 Ser-Asn
10 Thr-Lys
31 Asp-Asn
34 Ile-Thr
48 Thr-Ala
50 Lys-Arg
53 Asn-Asp,Lys
54 Asn-Ser
58 Ile-Val
62 Ile-Lys
63 Asp-Asn,Tyr •
67 Ile-Val
78 Val-Gly
81 Asn-Asp-
83 Thr-Lys
91 Ser-Gly
92 Lys-Arg
122 Thr-Asn
124 Gly-Ser
126 Thr-Asn •
128 Thr-Asn
129 Gly-Glu
132 Gln-Glu
133 Asn-Ser,Lys
135 Gly-Arg
137 Asn-Ser-Tyr-Asn
143 Pro-Ser,Thr,Leu,His
144 Gly-Asp-Val
145 Ser-Asn,Lys
146 Gly-Ser,Asp
155 Thr-Tyr
156 Lys-Glu
157 Ser-Leu
158 Gly-Glu
159 Ser-Arg-Tyr
160 Thr-Ala-Lys-Arg
163 Val-Ala
164 Leu-Gln
170 Asn-Asp
172 Asp-Gly
173 Asn-Lys
174 Phe-Ser
182 Ile-Val
186 Ser-Ile
188 Asn-Asp
189 Gln-Lys,His
191 Gln-Pro
193 Ser-Asn,Arg
197 Gln-Arg
198 Ala-Thr,Glu-Val
199 Ser-Pro
201 Arg-Lys
205 Ser-Thr
207 Arg-Lys
208 Arg-Gly
213 Val-Ile
217 Ile-Val
218 Gly-Trp
219 Ser-Glu,Pro
226 Leu-Gln
228 Ser-Gln
229 Arg-Gly
242 Val-Ile
244 Val-Leu-Ser
246 Asn-Lys
248 Asn-Ser,Thr
260 Met-Ile-Met
261 Arg-His
275 Asp-Gly
278 Ile-Ser
307 Lys-Arg
323 Val-Ile
327 Glu-Arg

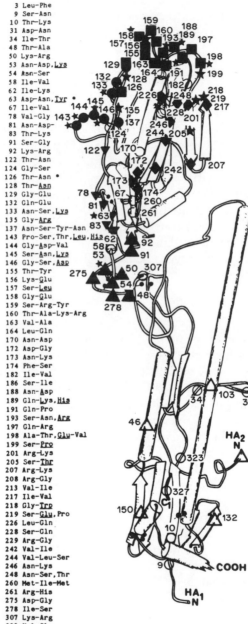

(b)

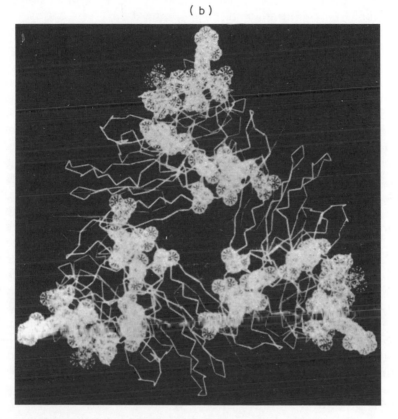

Fig. 6.3 Structure of the haemagglutinin of influenza virus. Natural variation since 1968 and monoclonal variants suggest the antibody binding sites on the 1968 HA. (a) ● = site A; ■ = site B; ▲ = site C; ◆ = site D; ▼ = site E. The symbols represent locations of natural sequence variation between 1968 and 1979. ★ = Single-site monoclonically selected variant—each star represents a separate variant; ★ plus site symbol represents a site of natural variation that has also been observed in a monoclonically selected variant. Underlined amino acids in the list of amino acid substitutions were observed in monoclonically selected variants only; no underline indicates in natural variants only; first letter underlined indicates substitutions found in both natural and monoclonically selected variants. An asterisk indicates addition of an N-glycorylation site; a minus indicates the loss of such a site. (b) Variable amino acid positions defining antibody binding sites surround the conserved residues forming the receptor binding pocket. The HA trimer is viewed from above; dotted spheres mark variable amino acid positions shown in (a). The centre of the figure shows the α-helices of HA2 extending 'into' the page. The receptor sites are inside the crescent of variable residues. Reproduced, with permission, from the *Annual Review of Biochemistry*, Vol. 56, © 1987 by Annual Reviews Inc.

The effects of antigenic shift can be mapped since the mutations that have occurred in various strains can be localised on the three-dimensional structures of the haemagglutinin and the neuraminidase.

The haemagglutinin of influenza A virus type H3N2 has been shown to be a trimeric homopolymeric protein (see Fig. 6.3). This structure has been derived from X-ray crystallographic analysis of the crystallised extracellular domains of the haemagglutinin. The protein is a type I glycoprotein (i.e. its membrane anchor is at the C-terminus) and consists of two subunits—the HA1 and HA2 fragments—which are generated by proteolytic cleavage of the HA0 precursor protein. This cleavage activates the protein to bind to cellular receptors and to fuse membranes. The major variation between natural isolates of the virus appears to take place in the HA1 fragment, which is generated from the N-terminus of the H protein and is the uppermost, membrane-distal part of the molecule. The membrane-proximal HA2 fragment shows less variability and contains the sequence of hydrophobic residues involved in membrane fusion. The mutations which have been found in natural isolates are localised in five areas of the molecule which have been named antigenic sites A to E. The three-dimensional structure of some of the monoclonal antibody-resistant mutants has been elucidated and this has indicated that the mutations which confer monoclonal antibody resistance alter the structure around the mutated amino acid residue. This indicates that the mutations alter the local structure of the molecule and that resistance to monoclonal antibody is not due to conformational changes elsewhere in the molecule induced by a mutation at a site far from the binding site. Interestingly, the resistant mutants were found to be localised in the same five antigenic regions A to E that had been determined by the analysis of natural mutants. These two facts together indicate that the mutants signify antibody binding regions of the haemagglutinin molecule as illustrated in Fig. 6.3. The receptor binding site of the HA molecule appears to be surrounded by antibody binding sites. This appears to be a general feature of viral receptor binding molecules. In general, the receptor binding pocket is placed below the surface of the surrounding protein so that antibodies are not capable of probing the inner structure of such pockets. This makes certain that those parts of the molecules which must be invariable to retain successful receptor recognition do not become altered under immunogenic pressure.

Similar observations have been made for the neuraminidase of influenza virus. The enzyme active site and the neuraminic acid binding site are in a deep hydrophobic pocket which has an inner lining of conserved charged residues. The binding site is not accessible to the antibodies and thus is free from antigenic pressure. Natural mutants and monoclonal antibody escape mutants are found to have changes in an area immediately adjacent to the binding pocket (Fig. 6.4). These residues appear to be in surface loops with high flexibility (see Chapter 4). The three-dimensional structure of influenza neuraminidase complexed with Fab fragments of two different monoclonal antibodies has been determined and shows that the area of contact between the variable regions of the antibody and the neuraminidase is indeed the area in which natural and monoclonal antibody escape mutations have been found. The interaction of an antibody molecule and the neuraminidase active site and the sialic acid substrate is of course determined by the actual three-dimensional arrangement of all components, which may explain the observations that certain monoclonal antibodies affect the enzymatic activity of the neuraminidase differently, depending on the type of substrate used. The neuraminidase of influenza virus is a tetrameric homopolymer in which four globular subunits are arranged around a fourfold axis of symmetry. This globular domain is linked to the membrane via a flexible stalk. Fig. 6.4 shows a diagram of the α carbon tracing of the neuraminidase subunit along the fourfold axis (i.e. looking down onto the top of the spike). The residues that are in contact with the monoclonal antibody are indicated in black and are shown to lie beside the entrance to the binding pocket. An interesting aspect of these studies is the observation that upon binding of the variable region of the antibody to the neuraminidase molecule, small localised structural changes occur in both the antibody (*paratope*) and in the epitope on the neuraminidase. These protein–protein interactions are thus better described as a handshake in which both protein molecules alter their structure, rather than as the lock-and-key interaction which was the original model. Thus, whereas it was once thought that the secondary immune response, involving somatic mutation of the antibodies, generates ever better-fitting keys, it now appears from the flexibility of the interacting molecules that mutations lead to a firmer handshake. The antibody molecule changes its conformation in such a manner that the paratope fits better to the epitope or that the amount of structural change induced by binding is reduced both in the paratope or in the epitope, as both changes do require energy. The structural change in the antibody, which involves the sliding of the V_H and V_L domains, may explain cross-reactivity of some antibody molecules to antigens other than the immunogen. The extent and the energy required to perturb the molecular structure of the antibody could be important determinants of the cross-reactivity of the antibody and may provide an even wider diversity among antibodies than that generated by light and heavy chain DNA rearrangements involved in antibody production. However, it must be pointed out that in structural studies of the enzyme lysozyme complexed to antibodies, no change has been observed in the structure of the paratope. Thus many factors such as the size and curvature of the antigen and localised structures of the interacting molecules may be of importance in the reaction between antigens and antibodies. The interactions of the two surface glycoproteins of influenza virus with antibodies

66

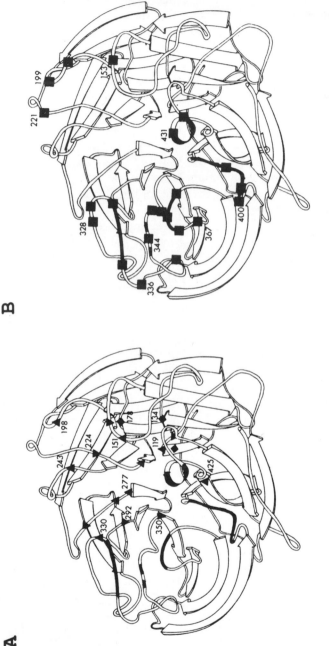

Fig. 6.4 Structure of the neuraminidase of influenza virus. Schematic diagram of the chain fold of the influenza virus neuraminidase viewed down the fourfold axis, which is in the bottom right position in both diagrams. Conserved positively charged (▲) and negatively charged (▼) as well as (◆) Tyr121, Leu134 and Trp 178 residues that surround the sialic acid binding site are indicated (part a) and seen to be remote from the variable residues (■) in part b. The 3D structure of a complex of the neuraminidase with antibody NC41 has been determined and the part of the chain that is in contact with the paratope of this antibody is shown in black. Mutations at positions 367, 369, 370, 400 and 432 abolish the binding of the antibody to neuraminidase, whereas mutations at 368 and 329 reduce the binding. Reprinted with permission from *Nature* **303**, 41–44. Copyright 1983 Macmillan Magazines Limited

are probably the most advanced examples of our understanding of this process. The analysis of the structures of the epitopes may lead to the generation of analogues via molecular modelling of compounds. This would allow development of vaccines that were not subunits of viruses but structural analogues of their epitopes.

INTERACTION OF B- AND T-CELL EPITOPES

T-Cell epitopes of viruses consist of linear peptide sequences from any of the viral proteins. They will probably differ for the various histocompatibility types present in the human population. Although many of the T-cell epitopes delineated for influenza virus are mainly representative of peptide sequences from the internal proteins of the virus (i.e the nucleocapsid and membrane proteins), some have been found to consist of sequences from the haemagglutinin. Particular peptides representing residues 306–328 of the H1 fragment have been found to be major T-helper cell epitopes in the human population, while residues 181–204 represent a major cytotoxic T-cell epitope. It is of interest that the T- and B-cell epitopes appear to overlap as the second of these two peptide sequences is localised in antigenic site B (see Fig.6.4). This is of theoretical interest, since T- and B-cell epitopes do not normally overlap. Some natural mutants of influenza virus have mutations in the major cytotoxic T-cell epitope.

EVASION OF THE IMMUNE SYSTEM

Parasites have developed very intricate mechanisms to evade the host's immune response, as will be described in Chapter 8. Viruses have a more limited potential in this area because they have smaller genomes and need to have surface structures that are specifically involved in recognition of cellular receptors. Nevertheless, a number of examples are now known where the viral glycoproteins are so heavily glycosylated, as for example is the case with the major surface protein of the human immunodeficiency virus (HIV1), that the host's immune system only percieves a 'cloud' of carbohydrate, which may be so similar to host molecules in an antigenic sense that the cover allows the virus to escape the immune system. Many of the natural variants of influenza virus HA have also been found to have accumulated mutations which affect the glycosylation of the molecule, and it appears that glycosylation probably masks a part of the viral surface structures in such a way that antibodies can no longer bind to particular antigenic sites. Similarly in mumps and measles virus it has been found that several monoclonal antibody-resistant mutants have alterations in their glycosylation patterns and thus it appears that one of the lines of defence of a virus against immune pressure is the glycosylation of the protein. It thus seems possible for viruses to evade the host's immune response by covering the viral surface proteins with carbohydrates or, as is the case for cytomegalovirus with β-microglobulin, a host protein which may provide protection for the virus as it is recognised as self by the immune system.

A further possible strategy for a virus is to suppress the immune system directly. In the case of the HIV major glycoprotein it has been discovered that certain parts of the primary protein sequence can act as immunosuppressive peptides. These may play a role in dampening down the immune response to the virus. There are thus many strategies by which microorganisms evade or hamper the immunological response of the host that has been infected. It is therefore necessary to be aware of the potential strategies that viruses may have developed to thwart the immune system of the host when vaccines are being designed.

SUMMARY

Viral vaccines in current use are primarily either *live-attenuated* or *inactivated* virus preparations. Live-attenuated viruses often elicit responses in both arms of the immune response and are therefore more likely to give long-term protection. Inactivated viruses are safe only in those cases when virus can be inactivated easily and effectively. T-Cell responses are often diminished when inactivated virus is used. This leads to the need for frequent revaccination.

The availability of high-resolution structure data has provided insight into the parts of the picornavirus virions that are involved in interacting with antibodies and have shown these to be areas of high sequence diversity. Structural information for the antigenic surface of enveloped viruses is only available for influenza virus. X-ray crystallography of the haemagglutinin, the neuraminidase and an antibody fragment–neuraminidase protein complex show that during binding both the antibody and the antigen change their conformation in a handshake rather than a lock-and-key interaction. Most of the epitopes in these two glycoproteins are conformational. Receptor binding pockets are in most cases sunken below the surface of the molecules so that antibodies cannot bind to them. As a result, they are not under immunological pressure. In the HA molecule of influenza virus B- and T-cell epitopes appear to overlap.

Some viruses and other parasites evade the host's immune system by masking antigenic viral proteins with carbohydrates, by binding host cell proteins to them or by containing peptide sequences within their proteins that suppress the immune system of the host.

SUGGESTED READING

Acharyan R, Fry E, Stuart D, Fox G, Rowlands D and Brown F (1989) The three dimensional structure of foot and mouth disease virus at 2.9 Å resolution. *Nature* **337**, 709–716.

Ada GL (1990) The immunological basis of vaccine development. *Seminars in Virology* **1**, 3–9.

Colman P., Varghese JN and Laver WG (1983) Structure of the catalytic and antigenic sites in influenza virus neuraminidase. *Nature* **303**, 41–44.

Colman PM, Laver WG, Varghese JN, Baker AT, Tulloch PA, Air GM and Webster RG (1987) Three dimensional structure of a complex of antibody with influenza neuraminidase. *Nature* **326**, 358–363.

Hogle JM, Chow M and Filman DJ (1985) Three dimensional structure of poliovirus at 2.9 Å resolution. *Science*, **229**, 1358–1365.

Rossmann MG, Arnold E, Erickson JW, Frankenberger EA, Griffith JP, Hecht HJ, Johnson JE, Kamer G, Luo M, Mosser AG, Rueckert RR, Sherry B and Vreind G (1985) Structure of a human common cold virus and its functional relationship to other picornaviruses. *Nature*, **317**, 145–153.

Wiley DC and Skehel JJ (1990) The structure of the haemagglutinin membrane glycoprotein of influenza virus. *Annual Reviews of Biochemistry* **56**, 365–394.

7 Bacterial Vaccines

INTRODUCTION

Bacteria are the cause of a wide range of diseases in both humans and in commercially important animals; experimental vaccines for the prevention of bacterial infections have been available for over a century. As a consequence of bacteria being complex single-celled organisms, vaccine design was extremely difficult in the early years of vaccinology. The rapid developments in molecular biology, immunology and biotechnology in the late 1970s and through the 1980s are beginning to have an impact on our understanding of the mechanisms by which bacteria and other pathogens cause disease. Individual proteins, appendages, carbohydrates and other cell surface structures have been identified and characterised and in some cases their role in pathogenicity has been determined. For example, *fimbriae* have been implicated in adherence of bacteria to eukaryotic cell surfaces, and the mode of action of many bacterial toxins has been better defined. The characterisation of individual bacterial antigenic structures has increased efforts to develop more defined bacterial vaccines based on purified cell components. Purified vaccines could lead to better quality control of vaccines, increased efficacy and to less reactogenicity.

In this chapter we will look at the complex nature of single-cell bacteria in relation to the problems of producing bacterial vaccines and consider some of the approaches that have been used to overcome these.

SOME GENERAL ASPECTS OF BACTERIAL VACCINES

Bacterial vaccines could be based either on live or inactivated cell preparations. Live vaccines were normally based on attenuated variants of particular pathogens which had lost the ability to cause clinical disease but were still able to establish a self-limiting infection and hence induce an immune response in the host. Inactivated vaccines were usually based on either whole bacterial cells or on crude cell extracts or cell culture supernatants. These cells or cell extracts were normally inactivated using either heating or controlled chemical treatment with reagents such as formaldehyde, phenol or glutaraldehyde. This simple approach allowed the development of a range of vaccines which varied greatly in terms of efficacy, safety and reactogenicity. Only a few of these became generally accepted for use in the community as a whole. Obviously the constraints on human vaccines were much greater than those for veterinary use. Table 7.1 lists some of the bacterial vaccines in common use in the mid-1970s. At this time we were limited to producing vaccines against organisms which could be cultivated easily in fermenters and laboratory medium. It was not feasible to make vaccines against organisms such as *Treponema pallidum*, the cause of syphilis, which could not be cultivated outside of the mammalian host.

Table 7.1 Vaccines in common clinical use for bacterial infections

Vaccine	Formulation	Infectious agent
Tetanus	Chemical inactivation of toxin	*Clostridium tetani* neurotoxin
Diphtheria	Chemical inactivation of toxin	*Corynebacterium diphtheriae* toxin
Whooping cough	Chemical and heat inactivated	*Bordetella pertussis* and *B. parapertussis*
Typhoid	1. Chemically inactivated whole cells 2. Live oral vaccine strain Ty21A 3. Vi polysaccaride	*Salmonella typhi* and *S. paratyphi*
Cholera	Chemically inactivated whole cells	*Vibrio cholerae*
HIB	PRP polysaccharide	*Haemophilus influenzae*
Meningococcal	A and C polysaccharides	*Neisseria meningitidis*

As we define the genes required for the growth and survival of pathogens in the host, we open up the possibility of creating attenuated variants of pathogens harbouring defined genetic lesions. The rational genetic attenuation of pathogens could lead to a new generation of live bacterial vaccines which are safer and cannot revert to full virulence. In the past the genetic basis of attenuation in live vaccines was undefined and it was impossible to control the quality of vaccine lots and to rule out completely the possibility of reversion to virulence. A good example of this is the tuberculosis vaccine based on live mycobacteria. Although this is a safe vaccine, great variations in the efficacy of vaccine lots have been reported in different parts of the world. It is possible that genetic drift in the mycobacteria during vaccine preparation is responsible at least in part for this variation between different batches. A new mycobacterial vaccine based on a rationally attenuated strain could eliminate this problem to a large extent.

Clearly we are in the midst of great changes in our thinking on vaccine design. Many experimental vaccines based on purified antigens or genetically attenuated strains are being developed. With any new technology, as we put forward new prototype vaccines unexpected problems are encountered as they enter the developmental and clinical stages of production. One common problem is our lack of understanding as to how to present defined vaccines to the immune system. Purified antigens have been found in general to be weakly immunogenic in comparison to complete bacteria. Whole bacterial cells contain a great variety of macromolecules and some of these have the ability to stimulate the immune system non-specifically. For example, cell wall peptidoglycans and lipopolysaccharides can act as adjuvants which improve the immune response to other antigens with low immunogenicity. For this reason crude mycobacterial preparations are included in commercially available adjuvants for experimental use. Unfortunately, many of the currently available adjuvants are toxic and are not approved for use in humans. Thus we need to learn more about how to stimulate an appropriate immune response to purified components, perhaps by using safe adjuvants.

At present many vaccines are delivered to the host by injection. This method has some practical advantages but it has drawbacks, both in terms of convenience and in scientific rationale. There have been recent efforts to develop vaccines that can be delivered orally rather than by injection. Oral vaccines which do not require the use of needles and medically qualified personnel for their administration would be of great advantage in developing countries. It is now recognised that many infections are acquired at or through the mucosal surfaces of the respiratory, urogenital or gastrointestinal tract. Perhaps as a direct consequence, the host has developed a sophisticated immunological defence system, known as the mucosal immune system, which represents a primary immune defence against invading pathogens. It is now well established that vaccination by injection is a very poor method for stimulating an immune response at mucosal surfaces. Mucosal stimulation requires presentation and processing of antigens by specialised cells at these sites. Interestingly, there is increasing evidence that mucosal stimulation at one surface is passed on to other distal surfaces via trafficking immune cells as part of the so-called *common mucosal immune system*. In real terms this means that stimulation in the gut can lead to the development of some local immunity in the lungs and urogenital tract. This further increases the attraction of the mucosal route for vaccination. Hence vaccine design for delivery to mucosal surfaces is quite different from that required for injected vaccines. Quite clearly, as has been pointed out elsewhere in this book, there are many factors that have to be considered when developing practical vaccines. Since we have now considered some of the general aspects related to bacterial vaccine development we can consider potential target antigens.

THE BACTERIAL CELL AND VACCINES

All bacteria exist as invidual cells with many typical structural features. The cell wall, especially surface exposed structures, and extracellular products are potential target antigens for vaccine development. Although the exact structure varies greatly between different pathogens the general features remain the same. Bacteria possess a cytoplasmic membrane which is surrounded by a rigid carbohydrate cell wall. The mycoplasmas are an exception in that they do not have cell walls, but they will not be considered further here. Gram-positive organisms have a wide variety of proteins, carbohydrates and other macromolecules attached to or associated with the cell surface. Gram-negative bacteria possess a cell membrane outside the cell wall, known as the outer membrane. Embedded in the outer membrane are a limited number of proteins and protruding from it are the characteristic lipopolysaccharide molecules present on all Gram-negative organisms. Mycobacteria are unusual in that they possess a thick, waxy cell surface composed of a heterogeneous mixture of lipids, phospholipids and carbohydrates. Many pathogenic bacteria possess distinct capsular layers, composed of carbohydrate polymers, which can be distinct zones separating the bacteria from the local substrates and environment. Bacteria can also possess a variety of proteinaceous surface appendages, either of defined or amorphous structure. Flagella are often present to provide motility through aqueous environments and within films. Smaller fimbriae and pili can be present in greater numbers. Fimbriae often play key roles in attaching bacteria to surfaces and cells within the body. The critical role of fimbriae in attachment, which is often a key early step in the establishment of infection, makes them attractive components for inclusion in vaccines. Bacteria also secrete or release a variety of molecules into their environment. Proteins and small molecules with toxic activity on mammalian cells are frequently released and are likely to play important roles in tissue colonisation by pathogens. They also release a variety of enzymes which have activity against eukaryotic cells and macromolecules. Bacteria produce surface localised and secreted proteins involved in gathering minerals such as iron from their environment. Many of these specialised molecules and structures which are essential for the *in vivo* survival of bacteria can be considered as potential targets for immunisation.

CURRENT AND EXPERIMENTAL VACCINES

A wide variety of the vaccines which are currently sold or are under development are aimed at preventing infections by bacterial pathogens. Many of these, especially those designed for veterinary use, are of dubious value because of their undefined composition, poor efficacy or high reactogenicity.

It would serve little purpose to discuss each of these vaccines at this point. Instead we will consider some of the major bacterial vaccines currently in use (see Table 7.1) and how modern methods are being used in attempts to improve them.

LIVE-ATTENUATED VACCINES

Commercial vaccines based on live-attenuated bacteria are very few in number. Various attempts have been made to introduce such vaccines in the past but many have fallen into disuse for various reasons, including instability and reactogenicity. Nonetheless, live vaccines can have many advantages and it is worthwhile considering why their use should be seriously considered, especially in the light of recent advances in genetically engineering organisms.

Live vaccines cause a self-limiting infection which mimics on a small scale the infection induced by the fully virulent pathogen. Thus in theory a live vaccine will produce most of the antigens normally expressed *in vivo* by the pathogen. This is important since pathogens may only express some antigens efficiently when they are growing in the host. Thus vaccines prepared from organisms grown *in vitro* may be lacking vital antigens. Live vaccines may stimulate immune responses in ways which closely resemble those detected during normal infection. This is an important factor because antigens processed during a live infection may be responded to differently from similar antigens injected as subunit vaccines. For example, live vaccines are on the whole better at stimulating cell-mediated immune responses than non-living vaccines. Live vaccines may also stimulate local immune responses if they are administered to appropriate sites, e.g. orally. This is because some live-attenuated bacteria may have the capacity to colonise mucosal surfaces and stimulate a secretory response.

However, the fact that live organisms are being given to a host raises the possibility that reversion to virulence might occur through changes in the bacteria or compromising conditions in the host. A live vaccine may be well tolerated by a healthy individual but the same strain may overwhelm a compromised host. These possibilities must be considered when designing new vaccine candidates. In spite of these potential problems new live vaccines are being developed because in some cases the pros still outweigh the cons.

BACILLE CALMETTE-GUÉRIN (BCG)

The most famous example of an existing live-attenuated bacterial vaccine is the tuberculosis vaccine, *Bacille Culmette–Guérin* (BCG). BCG is based on a *Mycobacteria bovis* strain originally isolated from a cow with tuberculous mastitis. The original isolate was extensively passaged on laboratory medium containing beef bile, apparently to prevent clumping and the accidental growth of the human pathogen *Mycobacterium tuberculosis*. Since *M. bovis* has such a slow growth rate the strain was passaged for a total of 231 times over a 3-year period! Calmette and Guérin observed a gradual loss of virulence for the cow and guinea pig with associated changes in the colonial morphology of the organism. BCG was first administered as an oral vaccine by Weill-Halle to children in 1921. It has subsequently been given to over one billion people, with a remarkable safety record.

The genetic basis of attenuation of BCG remains unknown. The initial strain was extensively passaged after it left the Pasteur Institute and was distributed around the world and further passaged on different media and in different growth conditions. Seed lot systems have now been introduced at vaccine production facilities and it has been possible to some extent to standardise vaccine production. However, it is likely that genetically variable versions of BCG are now made around the world and of course this will have implications for vaccine efficacy and quality control. New candidate live bacterial vaccines have recently been under field trial and at least one live human vaccine has been licensed in a number of countries in the last 10 years.

Hence the current BCG vaccine is a strain where the attenuating lesions are unknown and thus effective quality control of vaccine lots is difficult, if not impossible. With our improving understanding of the molecular basis of pathogenicity and the identification of genes and gene clusters required for the survival of pathogens *in vivo* it is possible to construct attenuated variants of virulent bacteria which harbour well-defined attenuating lesions. This approach has to be the standard by which new live vaccine strains are constructed. Defined attenuating mutations can be monitored using DNA analysis, the possibility of reversion to virulence can be minimised by using at least two independent deletion mutations, and the degree of attenuation can be controlled to some extent by choosing different combinations of attenuating lesions and strain backgrounds. Using these points as a guide we can now reasonably ask: how close are we to making a new generation of live vaccines? Many genetically defined attenuated variants of pathogens have now been isolated. These include mutants of many of the enteric pathogens such as *Shigella*, *Salmonella*, *Vibrio cholerae* and *Escherichia coli*, respiratory tract pathogens including *Bordetella pertussis* and encapsulated organisms such as the *Pneumococcus*.

TYPHOID VACCINES

Typhoid is still a serious health problem and the disease is endemic in many countries, especially in tropical areas. The existing whole-cell vaccine offers about 60% efficacy, although this may be lower for people from areas where typhoid is not endemic and pre-existing immunity to *Salmonella typhi* and other salmonellae may not be a frequent occurrence. The whole cell vaccine is quite reactogenic, hence the need to replace it with a subunit vaccine based on Vi antigen.

A great deal of experimental evidence has accumulated to suggest that live vaccines may offer better protection against invasive salmonellosis than the current dead vaccines. Much of this work was conducted using a murine model, although the data are supported by complementary information using other species such as cattle. Undoubtedly, inactivated vaccines do offer significant protection, probably due to the presence of systemic antibodies to *Salmonella* surface components. However, *Salmonella* pathogens can readily enter eukaryotic cells and survive for periods of time inside macrophages and related cells. Thus this location may provide an *in vivo* niche where individual bacteria can survive in the presence of serum antibodies. Some but not all live *Salmonella* vaccines can induce significant cell-mediated immune responses which may enhance protection. Further, orally delivered vaccines can stimulate secretory immunity which would provide an additional facet of protection. This type of rationale has prompted the development of live oral typhoid vaccines based on attenuated strains of *S. typhi* as illustrated in Fig. 7.1.

Early attempts to attenuate *S. typhi* relied on the isolation of mutants which were dependent on the antibiotic streptomycin for growth. Streptomycin-dependent strains could not grow efficiently *in vivo* in the absence of the antibiotic. One candidate vaccine strain was tested in field trials but the idea was not pursued when it was found that lyophilised preparations did not induce protection. This again illustrates the potential problems with vaccine formulations and presentation. Work carried out by Germanier in the early 1970s using the murine model and rough variants (lipopolysaccharide (LPS)-deficient) of *S. typhimurium* led to the construction of the *S. typhi* strain which became known as Ty21a. Germanier found that *S. typhimurium galE* mutants were attenuated and highly immunogenic, being able to induce protection against salmonellosis in mice. These *galE* mutants encode for the enzyme UDP-galactose-4-epimerase, which is involved in galactose metabolism. In the absence of the enzyme *S. typhimurium* cannot produce a smooth LPS molecule which is required for *in vivo* survival, since UDP-galactose is an essential precursor for LPS side-chain formation. In fact *galE* mutants are sensitised to the presence of exogenous galactose and lyse in growth medium containing this sugar. This may partly explain why *galE* mutants are attenuated.

Ty21a was isolated using chemical mutagenesis. As a consequence the strain picked up a number of undefined mutations and the molecular basis of the *galE* lesion was undefined. Nevertheless, Ty21a was found to be well tolerated by volunteers, and in extensive field trials in Egypt and later Chile there was no evidence for reversion to virulence. Initially, formulation problems were encountered with Ty21a but eventually enteric-coated

BACTERIAL INTERACTION WITH MUCOSAL SURFACES

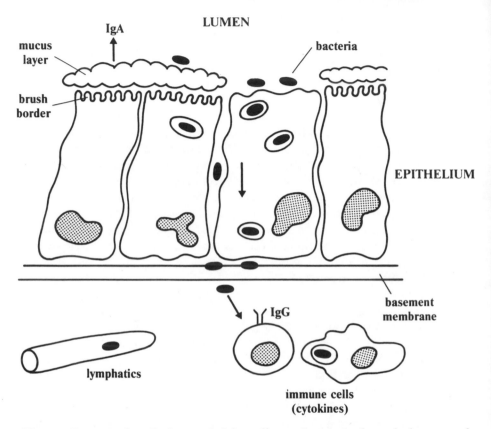

Fig. 7.1 Passage of orally ingested *Salmonella* vaccine strain through the gut and interaction with immune cells. Salmonellae cross the acidic stomach barrier and enter the small bowel, where they invade the intestine wall either via translocation across enterocytes or more likely by entering the gut-associated lymphoid tissues (Peyer's patches) through antigen-sampling cells (M-cells). Once in the tissue salmonellae interact with immune cells such as macrophages, which they enter. Salmonellae can stimulate immune responses in the host, including cell-mediated immunity (CMI), serum antibodies (IgA, IgG, IgM) and secretory antibodies released into the gut IgA. IgA antibodies may also be stimulated at distal surfaces, including the lung and urogenital tract. Some pathogenic salmonellae and vaccine strains enter the reticuloendothelial system (RES) and reach the liver and spleen, potentiating the systemic immune response

capsules were chosen as the optimal delivery system. However, further trials are now in progress comparing this with liquid formulations using sodium bicarbonate to neutralise stomach acids.

One problem with Ty21a is that multiple doses are required to induce acceptable levels of efficacy (50–60%). Thus Ty21a may be over-attenuated in some respects. A search for a single-dose oral vaccine still continues. A further important observation was recently made which is highly relevant to Ty21a. Workers in Australia used a cloned *galE* deletion mutation in Ty2, the virulent parent of Ty21a. This mutant was administered orally to volunteers, some of whom developed the clinical symptoms of typhoid fever. This work suggests that some *galE* mutants of *S. typhi* may not be attenuated and it is possible that other mutations contribute to the attenuated phenotype of Ty21a.

An increasing number of mutations are now being considered for incorporation into *S. typhi* live vaccine candidates. Most work has been carried out using metabolic mutants dependent either on aromatic compounds (aro mutants) such as *para*-aminobenzoate or purines (pur mutants). An *S. typhi* strain 541Ty was constructed by Myron Levine and Bruce Stocker in the USA which harboured mutations in genes *aroA* and *purA*. Although this strain was well tolerated by volunteers, immune responses were disappointing. More recently derivatives of *S. typhi* harbouring genetically fully defined mutations in *aroA* and *aroC* or *aroC* and *aroD* were constructed by Steven Chatfield in Professor Dougan's laboratory. A Ty2 *aroC*, *aroD* derivative was well tolerated in volunteers and was found to be highly immunogenic. These double *aro* mutants may be attenuated because *para*-aminobenzoate and other aromatic compounds are available only in limited amounts in mammalian tissue.

ORAL CHOLERA VACCINES

Many attempts have been made to develop strains of *Vibrio cholerae* suitable for use as live oral vaccines. Cholera is essentially a non-invasive infection of the small bowel. Release of a potent enterotoxin, known as cholera toxin, is responsible for the profuse watery diarrhoea frequently associated with cholera. Cholera enterotoxin is a classical two-component bacterial protein toxin. The A subunit is a single polypeptide of molecular weight 28 000 which has ADP-ribosyltransferase activity. The A subunit is delivered to the eukaryotic cell membrane by the non-toxic, highly immunogenic B component, which is a pentameric protein composed of five identical 11 000 molecular weight subunits which bind ganglioside GM1. Early attempts to make parenteral vaccines based on chemically inactivated cholera toxin were unsuccessful, although more successful work with cholera toxin subunit vaccines will be discussed later.

One approach to constructing attenuated *V. cholerae* strains is to modify the genes encoding the cholera enterotoxin. Mutants which do not express active A subunit are known to be attenuated. Early studies relied on chemical mutagenesis to isolate A^+, B^- mutants. Studies in volunteers showed that one such strain, named Texas Star by Richard Finkelstein in whose laboratory the strain was isolated, was found to be safe in volunteers, although a certain proportion of them developed mild diarrhoea. Texas

Star was quickly superseded by recombinant *V. cholerae* isolates where defined mutations were introduced into the chromosome using a mutated cloned toxin gene. After early studies using the A subunit deletion in different *V. cholerae* strain backgrounds an isolate developed by Jim Kaper at the University of Maryland, Baltimore, USA, named CVD103Hg-R was selected as a promising live oral vaccine candidate. CVD103Hg-R has a non-functional enterotoxin gene in the classical Inaba strain 569B. A mercury resistance determinant was used to inactivate the haemolysin of this strain. When 100 million viable organisms were given orally to volunteers over 90% produced bacteriocidal antibodies and these individuals showed almost total protection against diarrhoea upon challenge with the wild type parent organism. Side reactions were few and were similar to those detected in the placebo group. CVD103Hg-R and derivatives of it are now undergoing extensive field trials around the world.

Oral vaccines are probably more effective against organisms such as *V. cholerae* which colonise the gut mucosal surface. Secretory antibodies are believed to play a key role in controlling colonisation and enterotoxin action by preventing binding of the attachment proteins of the whole cell and the B component of the enterotoxin to receptor. The lack of efficacy of the whole cell parenteral vaccine is almost certainly due in part to the low levels of secretory IgA produced following vaccination using this route.

LIVE SHIGELLA VACCINES

Shigella species are responsible for bacterial dysentery, with at least two million diarrhoeal episodes occurring each year world-wide. The shigella species involved are *Shigella dysenteriae* types 1–12, *S. flexneri* types 1a–6, *S. boydii* types 1–18 and *S. sonnei*. The most severe disease is caused by *S. dysenteriae* type 1 (Shiga's bacillus) and certain serotypes of *S. flexneri*. Shigella causes invasive enteric disease with associated ulceration of the mucosal surfaces and release of blood into the stools. Mucosal immunity seems to play a vital role in protection against shigellosis and only live oral vaccines have shown promise in man. A variety of candidate live-attenuated shigella vaccines have been developed over the years. Most are genetic variants of virulent shigellae. Early vaccines, like those tested as typhoid vaccines, were dependent on streptomycin for growth but were unstable and therefore of little value as practical vaccines. Live vaccines based on *S. flexneri* mutants lacking the 220 kb pair invasion plasmid were found to be safe oral vaccines but required multiple doses to elicit protective immunity. Early vaccines based on *E. coli–S. flexneri* hybrids constructed using Hfr matings where chromosomal virulence genes were transferred to related but non-pathogenic *E. coli* were too reactogenic in volunteers.

Since we now know much more about the individual virulence genes of *Shigella* it should be possible to construct strains mutated in individual genes rather than blocks of genes. A starting point for this work may be an *E. coli* strain constructed by Formal's group at the Walter Reed Army Institute which is based on *E. coli* K12 harbouring the 140-megadalton plasmid of an *S. flexneri* type 5 strain and the *his* and *pro* markers from an *S. flexneri* type 2a so that the strain also expressed the type II and the group 3, 4 0-antigens of *Shigella*. At a dose of 100 million infectious units the oral vaccine elicited reactions in 20% of volunteers. This strain could in theory be further attenuated by introducing other attenuating lesions.

A further approach to shigella vaccine development is the construction of aromatic-dependent or *aro* mutants of *S. flexneri* by Lindberg's group in Sweden. One *aro* D mutant strain SF124 is undergoing evaluation in volunteers and in the field.

ORAL VACCINES AS CARRIERS OF HETEROLOGOUS ANTIGENS

Attenuated bacterial strains which can be used as live vaccines can also be considered as potential carriers of heterologous antigens to the immune system. This approach requires that the gene coding for the heterologous antigen is cloned and expressed in the carrier strain as a recombinant protein. In theory any attenuated strain can be used as a carrier so that the introduced or heterologous gene is expressed in an immunogenic form. An early example of this approach involved exchanges of chromosomal genetic material between different enteric bacteria. For example, regions of the shigella chromosome were crossed into *E. coli* and vice versa to create hybrid strains. A further development came when the shigella virulence plasmid was crossed into the attenuated *S. typhi* strain Ty21a. This hybrid expressed both *S. typhi* and *S. flexneri* antigens. It was well tolerated by volunteers when fed as a live oral vaccine but was found to be unstable. Different production batches showed great variation in immunogenicity in volunteers. It should be remembered that the expression of foreign genes, especially in high levels, in a host bacterium may be toxic to the cell. More stable variants which have lost the expression of the heterologous antigen will accumulate in the population and this is obviously detrimental to vaccine quality.

Attempts to use genetic engineering to express foreign antigens in attenuated bacterial strains have flourished in the past few years. Attenuated salmonellae have been an attractive choice of carrier for a number of reasons. They can be delivered orally, they have well-developed genetic systems for manipulating foreign genes and they can induce secretory, humoral and cellular immune responses when delivered by the oral route. A variety of antigens originating from bacteria, viruses and parasites have now been expressed in *Salmonella* vaccine strains. An example of a fimbrial

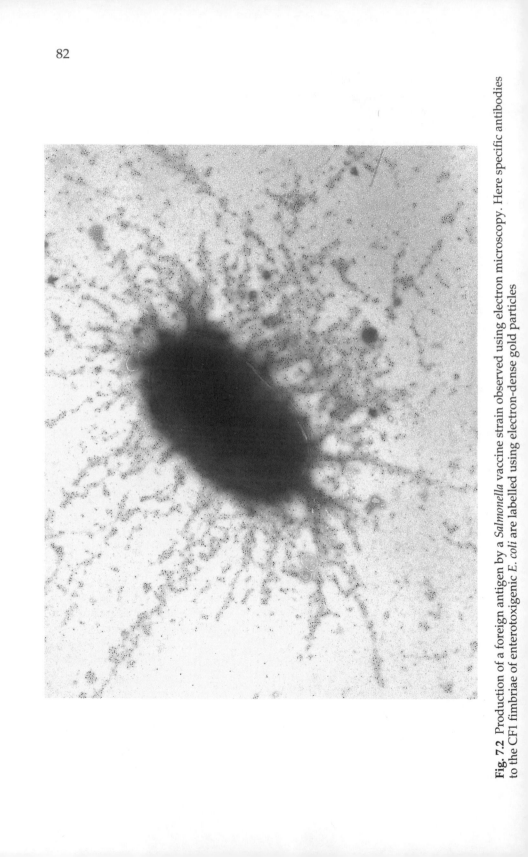

Fig. 7.2 Production of a foreign antigen by a *Salmonella* vaccine strain observed using electron microscopy. Here specific antibodies to the CF1 fimbriae of enterotoxigenic *E. coli* are labelled using electron-dense gold particles

antigen is shown in Fig. 7.2. Some forms of protection against virulent challenge have been demonstrated in model systems against toxins and pathogens, including cholera toxin, tetanus toxin, *Streptococcus*, *Plasmodium* and *Leishmania*. However, all of these are experimental vaccines and no hybrid vaccine other than those based on Ty21a have been tested in volunteers.

Other bacteria such as *E. coli* and *Yersinia* have been used as carriers. A great deal of recent interest has focused on BCG as a carrier. BCG is potentially attractive because it has been used safely in billions of individuals and is a strong inducer of cell-mediated immunity. Bill Jacobs in New York has developed a system based on modified phage for introducing foreign genes into BCG. Various antigens derived from organisms including HIV1 and tetanus have been expressed in BCG and immune responses have been monitored in model systems, and it will be interesting to see how the system develops in the future.

WHOLE CELL VACCINES

A number of vaccines have been developed which are based on whole bacterial cells. These, often referred to as bacterins, are usually administered by injection although attempts have been made to develop oral vaccines along these lines. Whole cell bacterial vaccines designed for injection suffer from the problem of potential reactogenicity since they are composed of a complex mixture of antigens, some of which are highly toxic for mammals. For example, the LPS of Gram-negative bacteria are pyrogens which cause fever and local reactions at the site of injection. In the veterinary field, a wide range of bacterins are produced. The number approved for human use is more limited.

PERTUSSIS VACCINE

The current whooping cough vaccine used in Europe, North America and elsewhere in the developing world is a whole cell vaccine composed of killed *Bordetella pertussis* cells. The vaccine inactivation methods vary but it normally involves mild chemical and heat treatment. Manufacture of Pertussis vaccine has to be carefully monitored since the growth conditions for *B. pertussis* culture greatly affect the antigenic composition of the cell surface and hence the immunogenicity. The antigenic variation of *B. pertussis* cells under different growth conditions has presented problems for monitoring vaccine potency. In the early field trials of whole cell pertussis vaccines there were significant variations in the efficacy of vaccines produced for different trials. A potency test was thus required which could be used to assess the potential protective index of different vaccine lots. Since whooping cough is exclusively a human disease no simple animal or *in vitro* test was available. The best correlation with protection was obtained with an intra-cerebral challenge in mice using a standard *B. pertussis* challenge strain. This test became known as the *Kendrick test* and it is still used in the quality control of vaccine lots.

Although the whole cell pertussis vaccine has proved to be extremely valuable in controlling whooping cough epidemics in vaccinated popula-tions, it has become somewhat notorious because of side reactions. Whole cell pertussis vaccine can be administered alone, adsorbed to alum adjuvant or in combination with diphtheria and tetanus toxoids (the so-called DTP vaccine). The vaccine is normally injected into the arm of very young, apparently healthy babies. Local and systemic reactions to DTP involving swelling at the site of injection and pyrexia are common and well docu-mented. These reactions could be due to any of the toxic cell wall compo-nents, including LPS. Some of the proteins such as pertussis toxin retain some biological activity following vaccine inactivation. In addition to these side reactions, pertussis vaccine has been implicated in more serious side reactions such as fits and brain damage. This is an area of great controversy and has led to the withdrawal of whole cell vaccine in some countries, such as Sweden.

CHOLERA AND TYPHOID INACTIVATED VACCINES

Two other commonly used whole cell bacterial products include *cholera* and *typhoid* vaccines. Again these are normally based on chemically inacti-vated whole cells cultured either on solid agar or in fermenters. Both cholera and typhoid are enteric infections, although the pathogenesis of the two diseases and the clinical symptoms are quite distinct. Success in vacc-inating against diarrhoeal disease has been quite limited in the past. Some of the problems associated with protection against mucosal gut pathogens have already been outlined. The requirement for local immunity involving secretory IgA means that *parenteral vaccination* is often inefficient. Probably as a consequence the whole cell cholera vaccine has low efficacy, with esti-mates below 50% being common. Both typhoid and cholera whole cell vaccines are also quite reactogenic.

The existing whole cell typhoid fever vaccine is under scrutiny because of its relatively low efficacy and reactogenicity, especially in areas where typhoid is endemic. As described above, studies using animal model sys-tems have suggested that live vaccines based on attenuated *Salmonella typhi* may be a more appropriate route to better typhoid vaccine development since such a vaccine could be delivered orally. Experimental evidence sug-gests that live vaccines may be more efficient at inducing cell-mediated immunity effective against *S. typhii*, although the exact mechanisms involved in protection are still being defined.

ACELLULAR VACCINES

Problems with whole cell vaccines have driven the development of acellular vaccines based on purified or semi-purified cell components. Acellular whooping cough vaccines were first introduced into general use in Japan. They were based on two defined antigens known as pertussis toxin (Ptx) and fimbrial haemagglutinin (FHA). Ptx is a protein exotoxin of *B. pertussis* which displays a variety of biological activities, including lymphocytoxicity and stimulation of histamine sensitivity. FHA is believed to be involved in attaching *B. pertussis* to the ciliated epithelial cells lining the bronchial tubes. Theoretically the combined anti-adhesive and antitoxic activity of this vaccine should induce protection against whooping cough. The Japanese acellular vaccine contains low levels of other pertussis antigens and is inactivated using chemical treatment with reagents such as formaldehyde. A formulation of the Japanese vaccine was evaluated in an independent field trial in children in Sweden. Although the vaccine showed some efficacy against whooping cough there, it has not yet been licensed for general use by the Swedish government. The calculated vaccine efficacy varied according to the criteria by which actual whooping cough disease was defined. The vaccine protected well against serious whooping cough disease but less well against infection by *B. pertussis*. Of course this in itself is not surprising. A serious fault with the design of the Swedish trial was that for ethical reasons the highly efficacious whole cell vaccine was not included as a comparison.

Since this trial, efforts have continued to perfect acellular whooping cough vaccines. New candidates include vaccines using improved methods of purification of Ptx and FHA, the genetic detoxification of Ptx using site-directed mutagenesis and the addition of new antigens to the existing components. The genetic detoxification of Ptx became possible after the cloning and sequencing of the Ptx operon several years ago. Ptx is a typical bacterial toxin based on the two-component model, where the A component has an enzymatic activity which is toxic to eukaryotic cells and the B component has a cell binding activity that is required for the effective delivery of the toxic A moiety. In the case of Ptx, subunit A is a single polypeptide with ADP ribosyltransferase activity. The B component is composed of five polypeptides, designated S1 to S5. The B component can bind to a variety of eukaryotic cell types and has mitogenic activity. Work to inactivate Ptx genetically has centred on the S1 subunit. Site-directed mutagenesis techniques have been used to replace individual amino acids in the S1 primary structure in regions that are essential for enzymatic activity. This work was guided by the fact that S1 has recognisable but limited regions of amino acid sequence homology with the equivalent subunit of cholera toxin. In the mutagenesis strategy molecules were constructed that harboured two separate inactivating amino acid substitutions to reduce to a minimum the possibility of regeneration of toxic activity by mutation during fermentation. Examples of inactivating mutations were the replacement of arginine 9 by lysine at the amino-terminal of the polypeptide and replacement of glutamic acid 129 with glycine.

One problem associated with manipulating the Ptx operon in *E. coli* was that the active toxin could not be assembled even when the complete operon was present. Even the S1 subunit was folded incorrectly when expressed as an intracellular antigen and at least one important conformational protective epitope was not formed. This meant that all genetically manipulated genes had to be returned back to *B. pertussis* in order to produce mutant toxin protein. This was not an easy process since *B. pertussis* is a fastidious organism with poorly developed genetic manipulation systems. Eventually, molecules were developed where the B component assembled with inactivated S1 subunit to form a non-ADP-ribosylating but immunogenic holotoxoid.

At least one of these engineered Ptx toxoids, the one engineered at Sclavo in Italy by a group led by Rino Rappuoli (Rappuoli *et al.*, 1991), has been successfully evaluated in phase one studies. Other Ptx preparations based on modified chemical inactivation techniques have also been developed. These modified toxoids can induce toxin-neutralising antibodies in the serum of vaccinated volunteers. What about other candidate antigens for inclusion in future acellular whooping cough vaccines? A number of surface and secreted antigens are currently being evaluated. One of the main problems here is that since there is no good animal model for pertussis infection, which is regarded as primarily a disease of humans, it is difficult to evaluate attempts to justify individual cell components. Work with true animal pathogens such as *Bordetella bronchiseptica*, which is closely related to *B. pertussis*, have thrown some light on this problem. Candidates include pertactin (P69), which is an outer membrane component of *B. pertussis* believed to be involved in cell attachment, the adenylate cyclase toxin and the fimbriae. The protein homologous to pertactin (P69) in *B. bronchiseptica* can be used to protect pigs against a disease of the turbinate bones known as atrophic rhinitis. Antibodies to pertactin (P69) can also be used to protect in animal models. Pertactin can be expressed in heterologous hosts such as yeasts and *E. coli*. The fimbriae of *B. pertussis* have only just been characterised in molecular terms.

Candidate vaccines containing different Ptx preparations and mixtures of antigens will be evaluated in extensive field trials. A serious complication of these trials is that any country which currently uses whole cell vaccine has a very low incidence of whooping cough. Thus a large number of volunteers will be required in order to obtain a realistic measure of vaccine efficacy. The trials would also run into ethical problems on the use of placebos and the rights of individuals to vaccination with a vaccine which is known to be protective. This is just one example of the ethical problems that appear when attempts are made to improve upon an existing and reasonably successful product, especially if the innovation involves a genetically engineered vaccine.

SUBUNIT VACCINES

A recent novel approach to improving the existing whole cell typhoid vaccine is based on the Vi capsular polysaccharide of *S. typhi*. Most *S. typhi* express this antigen, which consists of a homopolymer of N-acetyl galacturonic acid. Purified Vi antigen has been used in field trials in several countries, including South Africa and Nepal, as a parenteral vaccine. Efficacy equivalent to that achieved using a whole cell vaccine was obtained with a reduction in reported side reactions. Thus, Vi could be considered as a replacement antigen for the whole cell vaccine. One potential problem with Vi vaccination is that the Vi capsule does not appear to be essential for *S. typhi* virulence as assessed in human challenge experiments. Theoretically Vi-negative *S. typhi* would still be free to infect Vi-vaccinated individuals, although in reality this may not be a practical problem. Nevertheless, this highlights the growing trend to move away from undefined whole cell preparations to the more defined subunit vaccines.

Subunit vaccines are normally based on surface-located or extracellular bacterial components, although interest has also focused on some intracellular antigens such as heat-shock proteins or ribosomal proteins. One would expect immune targets for extracellular bacterial pathogens to be at the surface of or be toxins of viable organisms. However, for bacteria which rely on an intracellular niche to avoid immune surveillance, processed antigens from lysed intracellular organisms might be available for immune stimulation at the surface of antigen-presenting cells associated with MHC molecules. This possibility has stimulated interest in the heat-shock proteins of *Mycobacteria* which are strong B- and T-cell antigens.

BACTERIAL FIMBRIAE

Bacteria frequently express at their surface fimbriae or pili which play a role in attaching the organisms to surfaces in the local environment. In the case of pathogenic bacteria these are frequently the epithelial cells associated with the mucosal surfaces of the body. Fimbriae or pili are usually composed of homopolymers of polypeptide subunits with lower levels of accessory proteins which play defined roles in the adhesion process. Fimbriae can be detected using electron microscopy and appear either as defined rods or as thinner, more amorphous structures. They are often highly immunogenic and antibodies directed against fimbriae can directly interface with receptor binding.

Many attempts have been made to design vaccines based on bacterial fimbriae. There are two main problems associated with this kind of approach. Fimbriae are normally involved in binding to mucosal surfaces; thus systemic antibody is not effective as an anti-adhesive agent since it normally does not reach these sites in significant quantities. A secretory response is required to neutralise cell binding, so this has to be taken into consideration in vaccine design. A second serious problem is antigenic variation. Bacteria often have the ability to synthesise several, immunologically distinct fimbrial types. Antigenic variation can be generated by the bacteria using many different approaches. In the case of enterotoxigenic *E. coli* (ETEC), which cause diarrhoea, individual isolates express distinct fimbriae from different genes. For example, porcine ETEC isolates can express immunologically distinct *K88* or *987P* as well as common fimbriae. Bovine ETEC isolates express *K99*, *F41* or combinations of these fimbriae. Human ETEC isolates can express a wide variety of fimbriae. Some isolates have the capacity to express multiple fimbrial types; for example, the human adhesive antigen CFII has now been shown to be composed of three immunologically distinct fimbriae: CS1, CS2 and CS3. Strains express various combinations of the CS fimbriae and, moreover, the expression of fimbriae at the cell surface can vary under different growth conditions.

Other pathogens have even more complex forms of antigenic variation. *Neisseria gonorrhoeae* express pili which are highly immunogenic and have been implicated in binding these bacteria to epithelial cells in the urethra. Each individual *N. gonorrhoeae* cell harbours multiple copies of the pilin subunit gene in its genome, although normally only one is at a site where it is transcribed and translated into protein. Individual pilin subunit genes can be switched from silent to expressing sites by a process involving transformation with exogenous *Neisseria* DNA. Furthermore, during this recombinational exchange the transposing pilin gene sequence can be mutated— a process which increases the variation potential. An additional complication is that other *Neisseria* surface structures undergo phase variation.

In spite of these problems some vaccines have been manufactured which are based on pili. Good examples are the neonatal veterinary vaccines designed for use in cattle and pigs against ETEC. Porcine isolates of ETEC express fimbriae which allow the organisms to colonise regions of the small bowel not normally well colonised by *E. coli*. Most porcine ETEC types express one of a limited number of adhesion fimbrial types. These include a few antigenic variants of *K88*, *987P* and *K99*. Other adhesion fimbriae are known but these antigens are currently considered to be the most important and are responsible in part for the species specificity of ETEC. ETEC can also express defined bacterial toxins which can be inactivated for inclusion in vaccine preparations and these will be considered later.

K88, *987P* and *K99* can be easily released from the surface of *E. coli* by gentle heating to 60 °C and the released fimbriae can be concentrated and purified by various approaches. These types of preparation are highly immunogenic and antisera against the fimbriae will block receptor binding by the homologous fimbriae. Thus anti-fimbrial antibodies can also block bacterial colonisation of the gut if they are present in the intestine of infected animals. Vaccination against ETEC is possible in neonatal piglets and young calves because mothers can be vaccinated during pregnancy and anti-fimbrial antibodies in colostrum and milk will passively protect young animals which feed off vaccinated mothers. Thus this specialised situation in young animals allows the delivery of protective antibodies to the correct site.

There are few other examples where despite intensive efforts fimbriae or pili have been used as effective vaccines on a large scale. Problems associated with antigenic variation or inappropriate immune responses have compromised the approach. Some bacteria use several different methods for colonising cell surfaces and these can further complicate the design of vaccines. However, a number of experimental and veterinary vaccines based on fimbriae have been designed. A vaccine based on *N. gonorrhoeae* pili was recently tested in volunteers. The vaccine was administered parenterally but failed to offer significant protection. Other vaccines have been put forward based on fimbriae associated with *E. coli* that cause urinary tract infections but so far they have not come into general use.

TETANUS AND DIPHTHERIA VACCINES

Pertussis vaccine is normally administered to young children along with diphtheria and tetanus toxoids as part of the DTP childhood vaccine. We have already stated that tetanus and diphtheria vaccines, which are based on chemically inactivated and cell-free preparations of the respective toxins, are regarded as safe and efficacious. Can these vaccines be improved? The answer to this is yes—since multiple doses of vaccine are required to ensure good protection. The vaccines are manufactured using biological processes that are lengthy and run the risk of possible contamination problems, and the vaccines are not readily administered orally. Vaccination by the oral route would be useful especially in developing countries where it is desirable to avoid the use of needles to limit the risk of infection by agents such as HIV1.

In theory it would be desirable to manufacture the perfect vaccine, which would be a fully defined, totally synthetic, single-dose oral vaccine. We are a long way from achieving that goal for any bacterial disease. Since neutralising, antitoxic antibodies are all that are required to protect against tetanus and diphtheria it should be feasible to design a synthetic vaccine based on a few protective epitopes. The problem of vaccine delivery means that at present we do not know how to make such vaccines, and full antigenic structure of these toxins, even at the B-cell epitope level, is not defined. However, we are slowly moving in that direction. For example, genetically engineered toxoids for tetanus and diphtheria are already available and as mentioned in Chapter 5 an immunogenic diphtheria peptide had been identified 10 years ago by Sela's group.

A genetically inactivated diphtheria toxoid was first developed a number of years ago when chemical mutagenesis of the bacteriophage which encodes the diphtheria toxin gene was used to isolate toxin mutants which had lost ADP ribosyltransferase activity but were still antigenic and immunogenic. These mutants were known as cross-reactive material mutants or CRM mutants. One mutant known as CRM197 contains an amino acid substitution at position 197. CRM197 is being evaluated as a defined diphtheria vaccine and as a carrier for the development of conjugate polysaccharide vaccines.

Cloned fragments of diphtheria and tetanus toxins have been used to generate other recombinant toxoid molecules. Tetanus toxin is a large protein of molecular weight 150 000. A fragment can be cleaved from the tetanus toxin molecule using papain digestion. This polypeptide, known as fragment C, has a molecular weight of 50 000, is derived from the C-terminal of the molecule, is non-toxic but highly immunogenic and able to induce complete protection against tetanus toxin challenge in model systems. Fragment C has now been expressed at high levels in *E. coli* and yeast by Neil Fairweather in London, and the recombinant proteins can be used as safe protective antigens. The cloned fragment C gene is now being used as a basis to define the protective epitopes of this antigen.

POLYSACCHARIDE VACCINES

We have already mentioned an example of a polysaccharide vaccine based on the Vi capsular antigen of *S. typhi*. A number of vaccines have been developed or are under development which are based on polysaccharides. These polysaccharides are usually the capsular material of encapsulated bacteria. Polysaccharide-based vaccines have common features due to the unique immunogenic properties of polysaccharides compared with proteins. Our understanding of the immune mechanisms involved in the recognition of polysaccharides is much less than that of proteins. Polysaccharides are recognised as T-cell-independent antigens, as helper T-cells do not have a well-defined involvement in the immune response to them. As a consequence some but not all purified polysaccharides are poor immunogens. It is often difficult to boost primary immune responses due to the lack of effective T-cell memory. The primary responses tend to be mainly of the IgM subclass, with low levels of IgG and IgA. Infants under 2 years of age are poor responders to many polysaccharides—a serious problem since infections with encapsulated bacteria are frequent in young infants.

In spite of these problems polysaccharide vaccines have been developed and new approaches involving conjugation to carrier proteins are being employed to improve the immune response to polysaccharides. A vaccine based on the polyribosyl-ribitol-phosphate (PRP) antigen of *Haemophilus influenzae* type B capsule has been licensed for use in a number of countries. *H. influenzae* causes serious invasive disease, including meningitis in children. PRP vaccination has been shown to be highly effective in children over 18 months of age but is less so in younger children. Even children over 18 months of age produce predominantly IgM antibodies, the level of which cannot be reproducibly boosted. PRP has now become accepted, at least in the USA, as a new addition to the recommended vaccines for children.

Conventional adjuvants cannot be used to improve the immunogenicity of PRP vaccine. However, the carrier–hapten principle has been used to develop new PRP conjugate vaccines. The hapten–carrier approach was first exploited for bacterial vaccines in the 1930s. Conjugation of a small hapten molecule, in this case polysaccharide, to a carrier allows T-cell activation by the carrier to be exploited by the hapten. The immunogenic properties of a particular hapten–carrier combination will be dependent on several factors, including the average size of the conjugated polysaccharide, the carrier protein, the nature of the chemical linkage/spacer between hapten and carrier and the ratio of hapten to carrier in terms of weight. An array of different candidate PRP conjugate vaccines has been and is still being developed but vaccination regimes and assay methods mean that it is extremely difficult to compare different preparations. PRP preparations of variable average chain length have been linked to different carriers. Carrier proteins include tetanus toxoid, diphtheria toxoid, meningococcal outer membrane proteins and diphtheria CRM197. Spacer molecules such as the six-carbon spacer adipic acid dihydrazide are often used to link the polysaccharide to the carrier to improve stability and immunogenicity.

A conjugate vaccine developed by Connaught Laboratories using heated, shorter-length PRP linked via a six-carbon spacer to diphtheria toxoid has been administered to children in controlled field trials in Finland and Alaska. The vaccine is well tolerated and is able to induce in children under 2 years of age an IgG response which can be boosted. Younger children still generally respond less well to the vaccine; nevertheless even children less than 1 year old can make significant IgG responses to this antigen. A promising field trial in Finland suggested that the vaccine would be highly efficacious, although it performed less well in Alaska. The Connaught vaccine is already licensed in the USA for use in older children. Several PRP conjugate vaccines are expected to be evaluated over the next few years.

Other polysaccharide vaccines are either licensed or are at various stages of development. A pneumococcal vaccine based on multiple capsular types (up to 23 valencies) has been developed for prevention of pneumococcal infections. A conjugate vaccine based on the *Streptococcus pneumoniae* protein pneumolysin has been proposed. Vaccines against *Neisseria meningitidis* groups A and C have been developed but these have the same problems with immunogenicity, especially in young children, and conjugate vaccines are being developed. Perhaps the biggest gap in vaccines against encapsulated bacteria is a meningococcal group B vaccine. The group B polysaccharide is almost completely non-immunogenic in man and conjugate vaccines are being considered. However, fears have been expressed because the B polysaccharide cross-reacts with a related antigen in fetal brain tissues. This problem may take some time to resolve.

GENERAL PROBLEMS WITH ACELLULAR VACCINES

One of the main problems with non-living oral vaccines based on purified antigens is that few antigens are effective mucosal immunogens. Most antigens taken in as food are very poor at stimulating local and systemic immune responses. The body has obviously evolved to prevent unnecessary immune responses to food antigens that might eventually lead to allergies. Mucosal surfaces such as the intestine have specialised cells and immune structures involved in sampling antigens from the lumen of the intestine. For example, in the gut specialised M-cells take up antigen by phagocytic processes and the processed antigens are eventually presented to immune cells in the Peyer's patches which underlie the mucosal surfaces containing the M-cells. Exactly how the mucosal immune system discriminates between antigens is not understood in any detail.

It is known that the immune system can respond well to live pathogens which enter the body at or through mucosal surfaces. What about isolated antigens from these pathogens? Attempts have been made to identify and define the characteristics of antigens that will induce a significant immune response at mucosal surfaces. Two common properties including the ability of the antigen to resist proteolysis and also the ability to bind actively to receptors at the eukaryotic cell surface. These are both properties of bacterial proteins such as toxins or adhesins.

The best-known example of an efficient mucosal immunogen is cholera toxin and its B subunit (CT-B). Figure 7.3 illustrates the relationship between cholera toxin and CT-B. Cholera toxin is highly immunogenic when administered orally in very small doses (micrograms). Cholera toxin is also highly toxic and part of the immunogenicity may be due to local chemotactic and inflammatory responses. The non-toxic CT-B is also a good mucosal immunogen. Volunteers receiving CT-B orally quickly develop serum antibodies, the levels of which can be boosted with subsequent doses (see Fig. 7.4). CT-B induces high levels of circulating and localised IgG and IgA responses. Shortly after administration of CT-B, immune cells expressing anti-CT-B antibodies can be detected in the

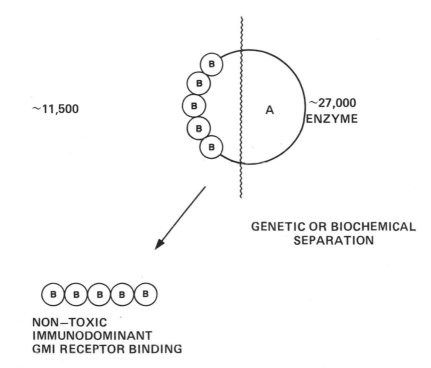

~11,500

A

~27,000
ENZYME

GENETIC OR BIOCHEMICAL
SEPARATION

NON–TOXIC
IMMUNODOMINANT
GMI RECEPTOR BINDING

Fig. 7.3 Diagrammatic representation of the isolation of the CT-B component from cholera toxin. The B subunit can be cloned separately from the A subunit or by biochemical means. CT-B is immunodominant and binds the GM1 ganglioside receptor

peripheral blood lymphocyte population. The level of circulating cells reaches a peak about 7 days after primary vaccination and these may represent a subpopulation of trafficking cells moving between different mucosal surfaces as part of the common mucosal immune system. IgA-producing B-lymphocytes may travel from the mucosal site of primary stimulation to seed secondary sites at distant mucosal surfaces.

A vaccine based on CT-B has been developed by J. Holmgren and colleagues in Sweden. CT-B is fed alone or with inactivated whole *V. cholerae* cells as an oral vaccine. Extensive field trials in Bangladesh and controlled trials in volunteers have shown that the vaccine is immunogenic and efficacious. The whole cell, CT-B combination vaccine gives better protection (50–60%) than CT-B alone. Protection is still present several years after vaccination but at a low level.

Attempts are now being made to extend the value of CT-B as an oral immunogen by chemically or genetically coupling antigens and peptides to the CT-B pentamer which is effectively used as a carrier for mucosal delivery. Success has been achieved with some hybrid molecules in experimental

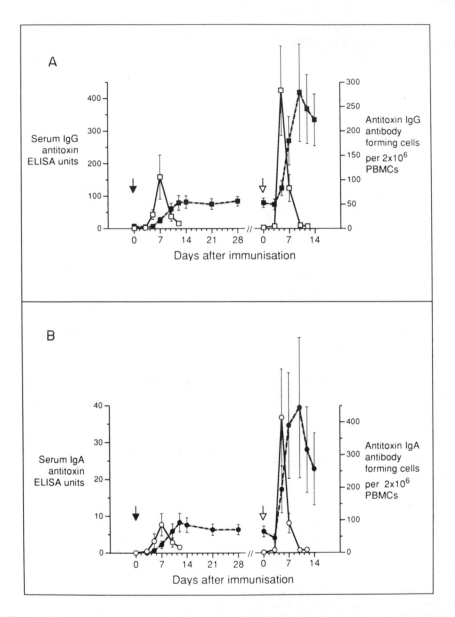

Fig. 7.4 Immune response to cholera toxin B subunit in volunteers administered a single or secondary oral dose of 1 mg (courtesy of Dr David Lewis of St George's Hospital, Tooting, UK). Volunteers were fed the B subunit following a bicarbonate drink to neutralise stomach acids, and the immune response was monitored on the following days. The solid downward arrow indicates the time of the primary dose and the open downward arrow indicates the time of the second dose.

Antibodies (dashed line) were measured in serum using ELISA, and antibody-producing cells were measured by ELISPOT, a technique that allows the number of systems but as yet no studies have been carried out in man. Cholera toxin itself and perhaps CT-B can be used as mucosal adjuvants stimulating responses to uncoupled bystander antigens. This has been achieved with antigens such as influenzae haemagglutinin in murine systems.

SUMMARY

There has been a resurgence of activity in the area of vaccine development which has been reflected in the field of bacterial vaccines. The move has been towards creating a new generation of defined vaccines based either on rationally attenuated, genetically defined live organisms or on subunit vaccines. There has also been a resurgence of interest in the oral route of delivery. This has been stimulated partly by the increasing incidence of HIV infection in developing countries and the potential hazards of contaminated needles. Vaccine development is a slow and expensive business and few new vaccines have reached the market. The haemophilus vaccine based on capsular polysaccharide is now licensed in the USA and is on trial elsewhere. Other vaccines are close to being registered. However, there is no place for complacency as we still have serious problems where no effective vaccines are available. An important area is that of diarrhoeal disease. The special problems associated with the development of these vaccines has been discussed already and hopefully significant breakthroughs are imminent. We have no vaccines which are effective against sexually transmitted diseases. This is an area where antigen delivery will be as important as antigen selection. Obviously there is much work to be done in the future.

SUGGESTED READING

Chatfield RN, Strugnell RA, and Dougan G (1989) Live *Salmonella* as vaccines and carriers of foreign antigenic determinants. *Vaccine* 7, 495–498.
Germanier R (1984) *Bacterial Vaccines*. London: Academic Press.
Levine MM, Kaper JB, Black RE and Clements ML (1983) New knowledge on bacterial pathogenesis as applied to vaccine production. *Microbiological Reviews* 47, 501–550.
Rappuoli R, Pizza M, Podda A, De Magistris MT and Nencioni L (1991) Towards third generation whooping cough vaccines. *Tibtech* 9, 232–238.

Fig 7.4 (continued) specific antibody-producing cells to be counted. Here numbers per millilitre of peripheral blood were measured. The solid line indicates the numbers of B subunit specific antibody-producing cells appearing in the bloodstream. Note the dramatic increase in the number of cells and the level of circulating antibodies after boosting. These circulating cells may in part represent gut-associated lymphocytes entering the circulation prior to seeding mucosal surfaces around the body. (A) IgG response; and (B) IgA response in this particular individual

8 Parasite Vaccines

INTRODUCTION

Unlike viruses and bacteria, parasites of vertebrates involve a number of stages in their development and often require a number of different host species. They have evolved living within close proximity of the immune system and have hence developed subtle mechanisms of avoiding or combating the normal immune responses. In this chapter, three major parasites have been considered and the approaches to vaccination discussed as they illustrate the general problems associated with parasite vaccines.

CRITERIA FOR PARASITE VACCINES

The nature of the relationship between the host and the infecting organism is generally more complex for protozoan and metazoan parasites than for viruses and bacteria. Like infections by other eukaryotic parasites such as fungi, there is a tendency towards their causing chronic rather than acute disease. This may be seen as a necessary compromise in that considerable time may be required for the parasite to develop from the invasive stage of its life cycle to the reproductive stage. During this time the parasite is potentially in danger of attack by the immune defences of the host. The evolution of immunoevasive strategies by the parasite in order to overcome these host defences is a complicating factor in the design of parasite vaccines.

The widespread nature of parasite diseases provides ongoing evidence of the efficacy of this strategy. As shown in Table 8.1 parasite diseases such as malaria and schistosomiasis cause a large number of deaths each year, but the number of infected individuals is vastly greater, with the ratio of infection rate to mortality rate being approximately 200 : 1 to 800 : 1. This is in contrast to that for bacterial diseases in comparable conditions such as typhoid, where the ratio is 40 : 1, or neonatal tetanus (1.2 : 1). Immunoevasive strategies generally involve either avoidance of recognition by the host immune system (either directly or by means of decoy molecules) or suppression of immune responses by secreted parasite products. A parasite may employ several mechanisms during its sojourn in the vertebrate host. Some of the better-characterised examples of this are shown in Table 8.2.

Table 8.1 Prevalence and mortality of some parasitic diseases

Infection	Infections/year	Deaths/year
Malaria (*Plasmodium* spp.)	800 million	1.2 million
Schistosomiasis (*Schistosoma* spp.)	200 million	1 million
Chagas' disease (*Trypanosoma cruzi*)	12 million	60 000
Leishmaniasis (*Leishmania* spp.)	12 million	5 000
Sleeping sickness (*Trypanosoma rhodesiense/ gambiense*)	1 million	5 000

Adapted from WHO figures obtained during 1977.

Table 8.2 Immune evasion mechanisms

Parasite	Location in host	Evasion mechanism
African trypanosomes	Bloodstream	Antigenic variation
Plasmodium spp.	Liver, blood cells	Intracellular antigenic variation
South American trypanosomes	Macrophage	Intracellular trypomastigote stage escapes from lysosome to cytoplasm
Leishmania spp.	Macrophage	Avoids intracellular digestion
Schistosoma spp.	Skin, blood, lungs Portal vein	Disguise as self Release of soluble antigen

An additional complication in the design of parasite vaccines is the size and complexity of many of the organisms involved. As *in vitro* culture methods are not generally applicable one must decide which antigens of the parasite are likely to be immunoprotective and then provide them in sufficient quantities for administration as a vaccine. This demands a thorough understanding of the immune responses induced by the parasite. For example, it has been shown in the case of infections by the protozoan parasite *Leishmania donovani* that the disease may exhibit a spectrum of pathology from visceral leishmania (Kala-azar) to asymptomatic infections. Overt disease is associated with *hypergammaglobulinaemia* and *hepatosplenomegaly*. Asymptomatic infections are characterised by skin test positivity to parasite antigens indicative of the development of cell-mediated rather than humoral immunity. Experimental evidence from murine models suggests that avoidance of the development of the pathological consequences of leishmania infection is dependent on the generation of activated macrophages capable of killing the intramacrophage stage of the infection (Table 8.2). A requirement for this is the stimulation of a subset of CD4$^+$ helper T-cells (T_H1) producing interleukin 2 (IL-2) and γ–interferon. These lymphokines can act synergistically to bring about macrophage activation. Should the other proposed set of T-helper cells (T_H2) be the predominant set stimulated, then the interleukins produced (Il-4, IL-5) act in the main on B-cells, leading to the production of largely ineffective antibody-mediated responses. The underlying mechanism by which either T_H1 or T_H2 CD4$^+$ cells are activated is not fully understood but is thought to be at the level of the antigen-presenting cell (see Chapter 3). With the above reservations in mind it is possible to delineate the criteria required for the development of parasite vaccines as follows:

1. The acquisition of a thorough understanding of the immune response to infection.
2. Selection of potentially immunoprotective antigens and their production by gene cloning techniques.
3. Development of delivery systems appropriate to the infection concerned (cf. leishmaniasis).

MALARIAL VACCINES

As shown in Fig. 8.1 the malarial parasite has both intracellular and extra-cellular stages in its mammalian host. The potential for protection by vacci-nation is demonstrated by the resistance which develops in individuals living in areas where the disease is endemic. However, such resistance takes a considerable time to develop, due, it is believed, to the antigenic differences in many of the wild strains of *Plasmodium* spp. In order to iden-tify immunoprotective antigens the strategies adopted by researchers have been either to examine sera from resistant individuals and determine the specificity of the antiplasmodium antibodies or to inoculate killed or radia-tion-disabled *sporozoites* (unable to develop into *merozoites*) into experimen-tal animals and then determine the specificity of the protective immune response which can be demonstrated by challenge infection. In this way circumsporozoite (CSP), merozoite (MSA), ring-infected erythrocyte sur-face (RESA) and gametocyte antigens have been selected as molecules with the potential to induce protective immune responses. There are valid rea-sons for developing vaccines from each of the stages of the parasite's devel-opment in its mammalian host. Thus the circumsporozoite surface protein (CSP) has been shown to be the only protein on the surface of this stage of the parasite. Monoclonal antibodies specific for it can prevent infection in experimental animals. Protective effects have also been reported following

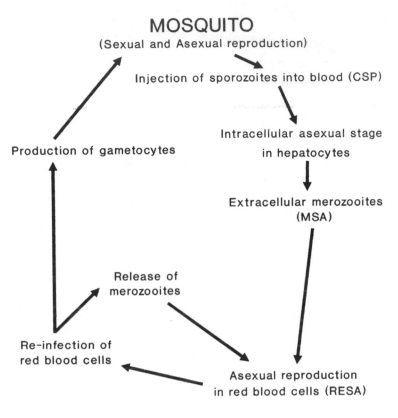

Fig. 8.1 Life cycle of the malaria parasite

administration of merozoite antigens and the RESA. The use of gametocyte antigens provides an example of an altruistic vaccine. The infected individual is not protected but transmission to the mosquito is prevented. This has the eventual effect of reducing the incidence of malaria in susceptible populations.

The analysis of malarial antigens in order to identify B- and T-cell epitopes has revealed that many of them contain an array of repeated short-sequence immunodominant peptides (Fig. 8.2). Analogous regions have also been found in the RESA and MSA antigens and are thought to be part of the immuno-evasive mechanism of the parasite. Unfortunately for the prospects of such regions as components of a subunit vaccine there is considerable variation in the actual sequence of the repeat region between

101

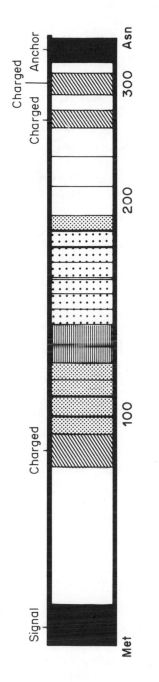

Fig. 8.2 Structure of the circumsporozite protein

different strains of *Plasmodium* spp., and the majority of human T-cell epitopes have been located in the polymorphic regions of the CSP.

The importance of T-cells as the agents of immunity has been emphasised by Pruihle and colleagues using sera from chloroquine-treated individuals from holo-endemic areas. These sera contain antibodies predominantly directed against liver-stage antigens and have been used to screen cDNA libraries and eventually select a clone containing an antigen present on the sporozoite and liver stage (SALSA). MHC class I restricted cytotoxic lymphocytes are believed to be the immune effector cells concerned with the liver stage of *Plasmodium* infections. As T-cell involvement in cerebral malaria is well established and associated with stimulation of the T_H2 subset it will be necessary to ensure that any vaccine designed to enhance T-cell reactivity is well characterised in terms of the subset it activates.

An alternative approach to vaccine production has been pioneered by Pattaroyo and associates in Columbia. Peptide sequences from several different antigens have been synthesised and assembled into one peptide. Field trials in South America have indicated that administration of the peptide can confer protection but it is considered that conditions in Africa may be more stringent. It is to be hoped that large-scale field trials in West Africa will be undertaken in the near future in order to assess the worldwide potential of this vaccine.

SCHISTOSOMIASIS VACCINES

Schistosomiasis (or bilharzia) is a chronic endemic infection by helminth parasites of *Schistosoma* spp. Infection occurs by penetration of the skin by the *cercaria* following contact with infected water. The schistosomules migrate through the circulation to the lungs and then to the liver, where they mature. The paired mature worms then migrate to the blood vessels of the gut (*Schistosoma mansoni*) or bladder (*Schistosoma haematobium*), where they shed eggs in either the faeces or urine. Some eggs may be found in the lungs or liver, where they become surrounded by inflammatory cells and their products to form a granuloma.

The prospects for the development of a vaccine against schistosomiasis should be good in that the infection is generally by low numbers of organisms and these are accessible to the immune system at all times. It is well established from studies on individuals living in endemic areas that resistance to infection correlates with increasing age. A feature of schistosome infections in experimental animals is the development of concomitant immunity. This is the state wherein the host harbours an active infection but resists re-infection by other schistosomes of the same species. An understanding of the underlying immunological basis of concomitant immunity would indicate effective vaccine strategies, and much research effort has been directed to this end.

As with malaria vaccines, the first step in the production of candidate vaccines has been to attempt to define the antigens inducing the protective aspects of the anti-schistosome immune response. Using sera from individuals living in endemic areas or from experimental infections in rodents, a range of molecules have been identified as being immunogenic. These have included integral membrane proteins such as Sm 25, surface antigens present during the early stages of the infection (triose phosphate isomerase) and enzymes essential to the detoxification of metabolic by-products, such as glutathione S-transferase (GST) Sm 28, Sj 28 and Sj 26. All of these have been shown to confer some degree of protection on inoculation into experimental animals.

A complicating factor in the development of an schistosomiasis vaccine has been the lack of a suitable test system. The rodent systems in general use are far from ideal, as a 40% attrition occurs in unimmunised mice between skin penetration and the lung stages. Some strains of mice differ in the structure of their pulmonary/cardiac blood supply, leading to differences in susceptibility. In humans much of the immune response is directed against egg-associated antigens, and the inflammatory response to these antigens is a major contributor to the pathology of the infection. As the rat is not a permissive host for schistosome infections—the full maturity of the fluke not being attained—it is also far from ideal as a model system.

Where animal vaccination experiments have resulted in the induction of resistance to infection the site and mechanism of this resistance are still debated.

Although a candidate antigen for use as a vaccine has not as yet emerged for schistosomiasis, much has been learnt about the biology of the parasite and immune responses to it. However, when a suitable antigen (or combination of antigens) is found, several formidable problems will remain. Not the least of these will be the testing of the potential vaccine in endemic areas. As these tend to be in regions where there are already severe demands on health care services, the funding of such trials will require international cooperation and altruism.

TAPEWORM VACCINES

Cestode parasites cause considerable economic loss by infecting domestic livestock and can also be of public health significance. The adult tapeworm is found in the intestine of omnivorous or carnivorous mammals. Cattle and sheep may form the intermediate host, being infected by the ingestion

---

of eggs (from the faeces of the final host) deposited on the herbage. These hatch to release the *oncosphere* stage, which penetrates the small intestine and migrates through the venules and/or lymphatics to their tissue location.

Immunity to re-infection develops after the primary infection and is maintained by the occasional ingestion of eggs. However, many intermediate hosts are not exposed to infection in early life and hence lack immunity. On chance exposure to infection such herds are extremely susceptible. As each tapeworm may contain 70 000 eggs a single infected dog can contaminate a whole field.

During the migration of the activated oncosphere in the intermediate host it is accessible to the immune system; antigens from this stage have been shown to be effective vaccines. The limiting factor in the application

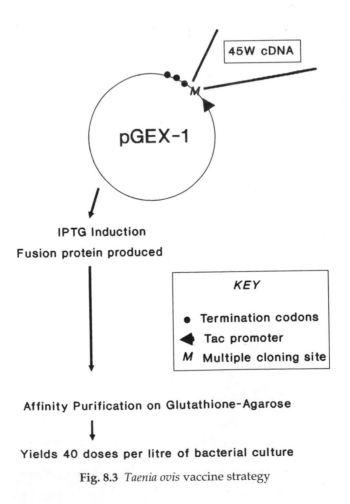

Fig. 8.3 *Taenia ovis* vaccine strategy

of such vaccines in the past was the lack of a means of preparing sufficient oncosphere antigen for widespread use.

Genetic engineering techniques offer a solution to this problem but they require the identification of the immunity-inducing antigens before the genes coding for them can be isolated and inserted into expression systems. Antisera from animals immune to *Taenia ovis* react in western blots of oncosphere polypeptides with antigens in the range of 47–52 kDa. Material from this region of sodium dodecylsulphate polyacrylamide gel electrophoresis (SDS–PAGE) gels was shown to induce protective immunity on inoculation into sheep. A cDNA library was made using mRNA from activated oncospheres and screened with an antisera to the 47–52 kDa proteins. Two positive clones (45 W, 45 S) were identified and expressed as β-galactosidase fusion proteins. Although inoculation with 45 W–β-gal and 45 S–β-gal fusion proteins generated antibodies which reacted with the native 47–52 kDa proteins, these were unable to induce immunity to challenge infection in sheep. As it was considered that the presence of the β-galactosidase element or the purification steps required to isolate it might have been interfering with the availability of potentiality protective epitopes, the 45 S and 45 W cDNAs were subcloned into a plasmid vector which allowed the production of a fusion protein linked to the GST from *Schistosoma japonicum*. Such fusion proteins can be purified by affinity chromatography on glutathione agarose, and unlike the β-gal fusion proteins do not require solubilisation in anionic detergents such as SDS. On inoculation into sheep the 45 W–GST protein (in saponin) gave 98% protection against challenge infection. As 1 litre of a bacterial culture can provide sufficient 45 W–GST to inoculate 40 sheep it would appear that the problem of producing a vaccine against *Taenia ovis* has been overcome. This strategy is illustrated in Fig. 8.3.

SUMMARY

The preceding overview of the progress towards the production of vaccines for three major pathogens has illustrated the problems besetting this area of research. It is probably significant that the successful production of a vaccine against *Taenia ovis* has occurred in a host–parasite system which had relatively few complicating factors when compared with schistosomiasis and malaria. The mechanism of resistance was well delineated and the immuno-evasive strategies of the parasite not well developed. One would expect that this successful application of genetic engineering techniques to subunit vaccine production might be extended to other parasites or to vaccines against their vectors. However, much remains to be done before a vaccine effective against malaria can be produced which will be capable of overcoming the antigenic variants encountered in the field. Nonetheless, a number of potentially immunoprotective antigens have been identified, cloned, administered to experimental animals and shown to confer protection. Of major current interest is the synthetic peptide vaccine against malaria which if successful will open up new vistas on parasite vaccines.

SUGGESTED READING

Ash C and Gallagher RB (eds) (1991) Immunoparasitology today. *Parasitology Today* 7(3), 1–66.

9 Possibilities for Future Vaccines

INTRODUCTION

It should now be clear that the field of vaccinology is at a turning point. We have gained a good understanding of how the immune system responds to the presence of antigens and have detailed molecular structures of the major pathogens. This information linked with the genetic engineering technologies has opened up novel strategies that should in the near future have an impact on how vaccines are made. However, for over 200 years, the public has been served well by the early inventions of Jenner and Pasteur and since then by those of many others, such as Sabin and Salk, and it remains to be seen if the new methods will in fact produce vaccines that will be any better or have a greater impact than the traditional approaches. Also there are substantial ethical, clinical and commercial problems in introducing something new as an alternative to an existing safe and effective prophylactic. Most traditional approaches depended on empirical methods, the underlying principles of which were quite unknown. For both the processes of attenuation and inactivation the early researchers had no knowledge of the molecular structures involved. Until recently there was no clear concept of the role of mutations in the selection of avirulent strains nor, in the case of dead vaccines, of the selective damage to or removal of the genetic or replicative material, which left the antigenic proteins relatively unaffected with regard to their immunogenicity. In the preceding chapters we have seen how the recent unravelling of the molecular structures of viruses, bacteria and parasites has led to a better understanding of what the traditional processes involved. However, as yet, this new information has not had a significant impact on the production of new or alternative vaccines against the major diseases, with the exception of hepatitis and pseudorabies vaccines. In part, this is due to the considerable success that existing vaccines have had, and only rarely do side-effects of vaccines currently in use catch the headlines. Commercial, medical and public confidence are all important components of whether a vaccine will be accepted, especially when the majority of individuals who are vaccinated are not ill and look to vaccination as prevention rather than a cure. Will, then, novel methods actually become accepted and new vaccines developed using rational design tactics instead of the empirical approaches of the past century? We believe that this is inevitable, and the design of any future vaccine will take into account the molecular changes and structures involved. It is very likely that new live vaccines will be designed rather than selected and that dead vaccines will be synthesised rather than inactivated. At the same time, novel concepts are emerging, which if they prove viable will revolutionise the delivery problem and open up new horizons not only in the treatment and prevention of infectious diseases but also in cancer and other conditions where a regulated control of the immune system can either prevent or cure an illness (for reviews, see Brown, 1990).

DIVA STUFF

IDEAL VACCINES

Before looking further at the new strategies that are currently being investigated for the development of vaccines, it seems appropriate that we consider again the characteristics of an ideal vaccine. Clearly, each disease will require a specific solution and not every characteristic needs to be present in all vaccines. Nonetheless, the concept of an ideal vaccine is one that has generated much tutorial-based discussion, and it may be worthwhile exploring some of the general aspects here to help stimulate further thought on the subject. For the purpose of this section we will look at two hypothetical vaccines: an ideal live vaccine and an ideal dead vaccine.

THE IDEAL LIVE VACCINE

The ideal live vaccine would not cause any disease or have undesirable side-effects, either related to the pathogen itself or to contrary reactions caused by contaminants. The vaccine should stimulate a high antibody response and provide long-lasting immunity. Few current vaccines actually do this and booster doses are generally required to maintain a protective level of immunity. In this regard, a wild type measles infection provides exactly what is desired by producing life-long immunity. This was demonstrated in the Faeroe Islands, which had been free of measles for many years. However, following the introduction of virulent measles during the 1930s, only individuals over 60 years old were found to be immune—in fact, only those who had had measles as a child. It is not clear, however, whether the current measles vaccine provides life-long immunity in all vaccinees, and revaccination is required, as with many other vaccines including polio and smallpox. From an administrative viewpoint, it is difficult in a complex society to ensure that everyone is vaccinated or maintains an immune status by having a booster dose at periodic intervals, especially as the circulation of wild type virus decreases. Hence there is always likely to be a pool of individuals who are susceptible to a particular infection and this makes it difficult to eradicate a pathogen completely. Nonetheless smallpox has been successfully eradicated, and current target viruses that are planned for eradication early in the next century are polio and measles.

However, the major problems in a vaccination programme are those of delivery rather than the efficacy of the vaccine. There would doubtlessly be advantages in having a vaccine that would spread naturally between individuals, producing immunity but of course not causing any disease. To a certain extent the currently used live polio vaccine spreads among contacts and helps to maintain a higher level of protection in the population than would occur if the vaccine was not able to replicate and infect close associates, although the problem of the rare reversion to virulence has still to be resolved. Hence we may wish to envisage our ideal vaccine as being able to spread among individuals in a natural way, successfully replicate in an individual, producing a high level of protecting antibody and permanently prime the immune system against its pathogenic cousin(s). If successful, the ideal live vaccine would supplant the disease-causing pathogen and would establish what has been referred to as endemic immunity. There are in fact many examples of this in nature, where harmless viral and bacterial agents co-exist with their hosts without any untoward disease problems occurring. In Chapter 7 on bacterial vaccines we have seen how attenuated *Salmonella* strains are being assessed as potential carriers for heterologous antigens because they can be used as oral vaccines to stimulate secretory and cellular immune responses in the host.

There would, however, be strong objections to our ideal live vaccine. From a manufacturer's viewpoint it would be uneconomic, as once released it would not be needed again. From the safety viewpoint there would be concern that the vaccine might revert to a wild type disease-causing agent. There would have to be world-wide confidence in the quality and safety of the vaccine. From an ethical viewpoint there are groups of individuals who do not want to be vaccinated for religious or other reasons, and some people who are immunosuppressed may show serious side-effects. However, it is interesting to note that although our ideal live vaccine may be a non-starter at present, even if it was achievable, many of its characteristics have been present in a number of attenuated virus vaccines that have been in use for many years throughout the world. Later in this chapter we will look at alternative strategies for the development of the next generation of live vaccines which may achieve some of the aspects of the ideal vaccine.

THE IDEAL DEAD VACCINE

Turning now to consideration of our ideal dead vaccine, we will first look at the advantages dead vaccines may have over live vaccines. In a number of earlier chapters we have seen that currently used dead vaccines are of two main types. They may be inactivated whole virus particles or bacterial cells, or be composed of selected parts of the pathogen, such as the surface protein or subunits which have been purified from infective cultures or are chemically synthesised or expressed by cloned vectors. The clear advantage of dead vaccines is their inability to revert to a pathogenic form. However, problems have been found in relation to the nature of the immune response generated which has not always given lasting protection, particularly since cell-mediated immunity is often not well stimulated. Similar arguments can be made against peptide vaccines, which in their simplest form would generate antibodies against a single epitope. Although in certain situations this may be sufficient to cause neutralisation of the pathogen, we still know little about the length of the protection period, and peptides representing non-linear epitopes are very unlikely to be efficient immunogens. On the other hand, the presentation of the complete or near-complete spectrum of epitopes of a viral protein can also be provided by using expression systems for cloned genes of antigenic proteins. This has been achieved and applied commercially for hepatitis B virus, for which the only vaccine available prior to the development of recombinant DNA technology was a vaccine prepared from the blood of carriers which is still used widely in the Far East. In spite of the success of hepatitis B vaccine which was produced in yeast cells, expression systems based on DNA technology still present problems associated with the purification of the immunogen and the potential dangers associated with stimulating immune or allergic reactions against residual host proteins.

What then of our ideal dead vaccine? The synthetic peptide approach seems by far the most attractive. A vaccine of course could be composed of a number of different peptides, each targeted to generate a different type of antibody, a number of which may be required to ensure a high level of immunity. In principle, this approach should be applicable to any pathogen—viral, bacterial or parasitic—provided we have sufficient detailed knowledge about the molecular structures involved in stimulating the appropriate immune response. The availability of such peptide-based vaccines could rapidly replace inactivated or subunit vaccines and could certainly challenge the continued use of live vaccines where there was any chance of reversion. Two other characteristics of our ideal dead vaccine are worth mentioning which would ensure their future popularity. We envisage that vaccines should be stable and be able to be taken orally. Unfortunately, as yet, neither of these aims has been achieved by synthetic peptides, but further developments in peptide chemistry or methods of delivery (see later) may make delivery by the oral route possible. Finally, synthetic vaccines will require a highly sophisticated understanding of both the molecular structures of the pathogen and the detailed pathways of the immune response. They will be expensive, but their safety margins will make them attractive to industry as well as to the general public, at least in developed countries. The question remains as to whether they will be affordable to the less developed countries, where the prevention of infectious diseases requires major health care and social programmes.

Associated with severe malnutrition, it is perhaps important to recall that a child dies of measles every 20 seconds. Unfortunately, the currently available measles vaccine is thermally labile and requires refrigeration throughout the long period of transportation and until just prior to inoculation.

One feature that is essential for the exploitation of dead or synthetic vaccines is how to enhance both arms of the immune response. We will now look at exciting new ways of presenting antigens that could revolutionise the use of synthetic immunogens.

IMMUNOSTIMULATING COMPLEXES

As a general rule, several copies of an antigen should be presented to the immune system to generate the optimal response. Most synthetic antigens or purified surface components will be in a monomeric state, and over many years techniques have been developed which enhance the immune response, i.e. the use of adjuvants. The immunostimulating complex or iscom is a more recent development which enhances both the antibody-mediated and cell-mediated immunity, including the induction of cytotoxic T-cells.

The iscom is an adjuvant particle onto which a number of copies of the antigen are attached. The active substance in the iscom is Quil A, which is extracted from the bark of the South American tree *Quilaja saponaria molina*. As well as Quil A, an iscom will contain cholesterol and phosphatidyl choline, a less rigid lipid, and the antigen in equimolar amounts. As hydrophobic interactions hold the constituents together, membrane proteins, with their transmembrane domains, have initially been the antigens of choice for incorporation into iscoms. Iscom formation is dependent upon the specific binding between Quil A and cholesterol, and electron micrographs show that spherical cage-like structures form, even in the absence of antigen, with a mean diameter of about 40 nm, made up of 12 nm morphological units.

As seen in Chapter 3, the early fate of antigen upon administration is of great importance for the subsequent induction of the immune response. Antigen must enter the pathway for immune stimulation and iscoms enhance their uptake by presenting cells. Of considerable interest is the observation that iscoms can induce an efficient serum antibody response following intranasal application as well as by parenteral immunisation. With influenza surface proteins iscoms also induce cytotoxic T-memory cells, which is desirable in a vaccine as that is the way in which the infected individual clears virus-infected cells. The surface proteins of over 20 different enveloped viruses have been included in iscoms and all have their immunogenicity greatly enhanced, with some tenfold higher levels of serum antibody responses than found with antigens presented in micelles or in intact virus particles. Recent studies show that synthetic peptides can also be integrated into iscoms provided they have an accessible hydrophobic region. In general, carrier molecules such as the HA protein of influenza are used to provide the T-cell epitope required to ensure that an antibody response is elicited.

The application and progress of iscoms to vaccination has been extensively reviewed by Morein *et al.* (1990). Their ability to enhance the immune response will clearly have a major influence in the development of future vaccines.

ANTI-IDIOTYPIC VACCINES

Neither the synthetic peptide nor recombinant DNA approaches can deal with antigens which are based on non-protein substances, such as lipid, carbohydrate or glycolipid. Another approach, which is based on our increased knowledge of the immune system and the nature of antibodies themselves, is known as anti-idiotypic vaccination. Antibody molecules, discussed briefly in Chapter 3, are large immunoglobulins which have many properties in common, but each antibody molecule is characterised by a specific antigen binding site, often referred to as the idiotypic determinant (Id) or idiotype which is located in the variable (V) region. Antibodies raised against a specific idiotype (anti-idiotype) can mimic the conformation and shape of the primary antigen of an infecting agent even if this is lipid, carbohydrate or glycolipid in nature. Anti-Id antibodies can therefore be used to stimulate an immune response against a foreign antigen. The development of anti-idiotypic vaccines is still at an early stage but one attractive strategy illustrates how they may be used to produce the functional state of an epitope in a peptide-based form. Hybridomas producing monoclonal anti-idiotypes can be obtained and subsequently homogeneous immunoglobulin mRNA purified and the sequence around the V region of the immunoglobulin determined by standard sequencing methods (see Chapter 2). Knowledge of the amino acid sequence of the anti-idiotype should allow the production of synthetic anti-Id preparations by use of either recombinant DNA or peptide-based technologies.

GENETICALLY ENGINEERED LIVE VACCINES

As we have seen, the advent of recombinant DNA technologies opened up new ways of manipulating genetic material, and prokaryotic cells and viruses have provided much of the stimulus for these developments. Over the last 10–20 years an immense amount of information about the genetic make-up of pathogenic organisms has accumulated, and numerous attempts are now being made to exploit this by the construction of hybrid agents that could be useful as vaccines.

LIVE BACTERIAL VACCINES

Recent developments in the use of bacteria as vectors for carrying foreign antigens has been described in Chapter 7 and will not be discussed further here.

VACCINIA RECOMBINANTS

The successful use of vaccinia virus for the eradication of smallpox led Moss and Paoletti and their colleagues in 1982 to the idea of using genetically engineered live virus as a vector for carrying foreign antigens as a strategy in future vaccination programmes. To date, over 100 different vaccinia virus recombinants have been described and many of them can protect animals against challenge with the appropriate pathogen. For example, an HIV1–vaccinia recombinant has already been tested in humans and induces a response to the HIV1 envelope glycoprotein. Success of current field trials with vaccinia recombinants expressing rabies virus glycoproteins may lead to widespread use of recombinants as animal vaccines, as it has already been shown that recombinants expressing the rabies virus glycoprotein protect foxes and racoons against challenge with rabies virus even when the virus used to immunise is left in baited food.

The construction of vaccinia virus recombinants has proven to be a relatively straightforward matter, depending upon the intracellular homologous recombination between vaccinia virus DNA and especially engineered plasmids. For example, a plasmid is constructed which has the required foreign gene (X) adjacent to a vaccinia gene promoter (P). This arrangement (P–X) is flanked by vaccinia thymidine kinase sequences (TK_L and TK_R). Following homologous recombination at the TK_L and TK_R sites, the foreign gene together with the vaccinia virus promoter are inserted into the vaccinia virus DNA. Subsequent replication and packaging of the recombinant DNA takes place to give live recombinant virus. Selection of the recombinant virus can use the fact that the recombinants will have a TK minus phenotype and will contain sequences corresponding to the foreign gene (X).

Many virus genes have been expressed by vaccinia recombinants and these have been summarised by Mackett in his excellent review 'Vaccinia virus as a vector' (1990). The level of expression of the foreign gene is greatly influenced by the promoter used, and up to 1–2 mg of foreign protein per litre of infected cell culture has been obtained. An important feature in regard to vaccination is that the foreign expressed protein appears to undergo normal post-translation modifications such as glycosylation and proteolytic cleavage and are also transported normally to appropriate sub-cellular sites. For example, the influenza A virus haemagglutinin migrates to the apical surface of the recombinant infected cell, whereas murine leukaemia and vesicular stomatitis virus envelope proteins move to the basolateral surface of cells.

It is likely that many of the features that made vaccinia virus such an effective vaccine against smallpox will be retained by recombinant vaccinia viruses. Such vaccines would be cheap to manufacture and administer. They would be stable and not require refrigeration. Also, like naturally occurring pathogens, they effectively stimulate both antibody and cell-mediated immune responses. Furthermore, the large size of the virus genome enables the accommodation of a number of foreign genes, and the construction of polyvalent vaccines to suit the specific needs of certain geo-graphical areas is possible. For example, as suggested by Mackett (1990), a vaccine that simultaneously immunised against hepatitis B virus, Epstein–Barr virus, poliovirus and several haemorrhagic fevers would be highly desirable in southern China.

In conclusion, research during the past 10 years has opened up new strategies for future vaccines based on using vaccinia or similar large virus-es from the pox family as vectors for carrying foreign antigens. However, as mentioned above, there are genuine grounds for concern that recombi-nants may have altered tropisms or pathogenicity. They may be spread across different species or recombination between other pox viruses, per-haps generating novel diseases. All these are real questions that require close scrutiny prior to wide-scale use of these new live agents. However, the questions and the problems are no different from those faced during the introduction of earlier live vaccines, from Jenner's use of cowpox in 1796 to the more sophisticated attenuation of poliovirus by Sabin during the 1950s. In the final analysis the only way to assess a recombinant will be large-scale clinical trials, the acceptability of which will greatly depend on how serious the disease problem is perceived to be.

As in most parts of the world vaccination against smallpox continued until about 10 years ago, the use of vaccinia virus recombinants for human vaccination may be limited at present as the immune status of individuals may decrease the immune response to the foreign gene. However, in geo-graphic regions where diseases causing high morbidity and mortality greatly outweigh the rare adverse complications, vaccinia virus recombi-nants provide an attractive alternative to current methods of control. Of greater current interest is the potential widespread use of these engineered vaccines for animal diseases, such as rabies and pseudorabies. This prospect will test considerably the environmental and regulatory issues raised, not only at local but also at international levels, and requires a con-siderable increase in our knowledge about the spread of vaccinia virus among wild and domestic animal species.

Despite obvious difficulties and concerns, the strategy of using vaccinia and other pox viruses as vectors, established over the last 10 years, will influence the development of vaccines for many years to come.

PICORNAVIRUS VECTORS

In addition to the pox group discussed above, which are very large viruses with the capacity to code for over 100 different proteins, a number of other viruses have been considered as vectors for carrying foreign antigen, including adenovirus, herpesvirus and baculoviruses. In contrast, picornaviruses are among the smallest viruses known and contain only seven or eight genes. As described in Chapter 6, knowledge of the molecular structure of a number of picornaviruses, including poliovirus, rhinovirus, foot-and-mouth disease virus (FMDV) and bovine enterovirus (BEV), has led to a detailed understanding of the importance of specific epitopes for the stimulation of an immune response. Since the early 1980s, major advances have been achieved by Jeffrey Almond's, Eckard Wimmer's and Marc Girard's groups in the construction of poliovirus chimeras, and the results have been sufficiently successful to encourage others to entertain the possibility of exploiting different picornaviruses as potential vectors for both animal and human vaccines (see Almond and Burke, 1990).

In contrast to the strategy involved in the construction of vaccinia virus recombinants, where whole foreign genes are inserted, the aim of the picornavirus approach is to be highly selective and insert only the minimal amino acid sequence that will stimulate the required immune response. The possibility also exists of deleting a host antigenic site and inserting a foreign epitope in its place, hence conserving the size of the genome of the new hybrid virus, which is required for efficient replication and spread.

The strategy used in making these chimeric constructs depends on the fact that picornavirus RNA is infectious and is able to function as a messenger RNA for the production of viral protein. Consequently, it was to be expected that a full-length cDNA clone of a picornavirus, transfected into a mammalian cell, would be transcribed into viral RNA and translated into viral protein. The viral RNA would subsequently be replicated and infectious virus particles produced. This possibility was first shown to be feasible by Racaniello and Baltimore in 1981, allowing the full application of recombinant DNA techniques to the manipulation of picornavirus genomes. More recently, the construction of cassette vectors in which specific and unique restriction endonuclease sites are engineered into cDNA at positions flanking the desired insertion site has greatly facilitated the production of a wide range of chimeric viruses.

The first practical demonstration of this approach was achieved with the Sabin poliovirus vaccine strains by the successful transfer of the antigenic site 1 of serotype 3 strain into serotype 1 strain. The resulting intertypic chimeras displayed antigenic and immunogenic characteristics of both types 1 and 3 viruses. The construction of a type 1 Sabin strain expressing the type 3 antigenic site has considerable implications for vaccination against poliomyelitis, as the major risks involved in current vaccination programmes are caused by type 3 whereas type 1 is probably the safest live vaccine ever used in humans. Parts of numerous other foreign antigens have been inserted into poliovirus, including a well-characterised epitope from the transmembrane protein gp41 of HIV1 and a 16 amino acid segment of the major capsid protein of human papillomavirus, which is considered to be associated with the development of carcinoma of the cervix. These studies have recently been reviewed by Almond and Burke (1990). A large number of the constructs have been shown to produce viable viruses which are capable of stimulating antibody responses. The longest sequence inserted so far is 21 amino acids although occasionally even shorter sequences seem to destroy the viability of the virus. Of course many epitopes involve complex conformational structures rather than a short single unique amino acid sequence and it has not yet been possible to introduce these more complex inserts and retain both antigenic integrity and viability of the chimeric virus.

Of particular interest to the authors is the possibility of using a harmless BEV as a vector for carrying the antigenic sites of FMDV or other animal pathogens such as liver fluke (*Fasciola hepatica*). Our concept is different from using an existing vaccine such as the Sabin polio vaccine, but involves making use of a virus that is naturally occurring in domestic populations and although endemic in the community does not appear to cause any significant disease. Like many apparently harmless viruses that are known to infect man such as ECHO viruses, BEV appears to be epizootic in cattle herds, infects calves and replicates and stimulates an immune status in most adult cattle. The exploitation of these harmless agents as vectors could open up a new avenue of controlling infectious diseases.

The incorporation of the FMDV peptide described in Chapter 5 would involve the introduction of only 63 nucleotides into the BEV genome, and hence the 'BEV–FMDV' chimera would not contain any of the potential FMDV pathogenic causing factors. Furthermore, should the BEV–FMDV hybrid vaccine behave in the field as the naturally occurring BEV does, it should become established as an endemic agent. It has been mentioned above that one of the advantages of a live virus vaccine is that there is nearly always an element of what is called 'herd immunity' as the vaccine can be passed on to neighbours in the herd or close associates in family or school. The concept of endemic immunity introduces the idea that the vaccine would be retained in the population and passed not only horizontally within a herd, for example during one season, but would be passed vertically to new generations of animals in the same way as apparently occurs with BEV.

In considering the potential of such a BEV–FMDV chimera, this is essentially an alternative method of presenting the FMDV peptide discussed in Chapter 5. Rather than making the peptide synthetically (chemically), the peptide sequence and structure would be generated in the field during the replication of the virus in the infected (vaccinated) animals. Such a vaccine(s) would be cheaper and could be extremely effective in controlling, if not eradicating, diseases in wild as well as domestic animals.

However, serious concern surrounds the question of the construction of any novel agent and, prior to release into the environment, adequate assessments must be made of the potential risks, which may involve a change in host range or the pathogenicity of the chimeras. One major advantage of considering picornaviruses as vectors is their relative simplicity and the likelihood that within the foreseeable future sufficient knowledge of the detailed molecular structure will allow very precise information about the nature of not only immunogenic sites but also receptor binding sites and various other sites that influence the host range, pathogenicity or neurovirulence of the virus. When more molecular information becomes available, vaccinologists can approach the construction of what may well be the nearest we will come to our ideal vaccine, with much more confidence than at present.

CONCLUSIONS

For over a century the technology of vaccination has been the mainstay of our fight against infectious diseases, especially those caused by viruses. Of course in the mid-1900s the discovery of antibiotics revolutionised treatment of bacterial diseases, and subsequently a great deal of attention has been given to the search for chemotherapeutic agents against viruses. Unfortunately, this search has been only partially successful and the relatively rapid rate of mutation, especially among the RNA viruses, together with the fact that most antiviral agents act after infection of target cells has taken place and while replication is underway, allows the evolution of resistant forms at an unacceptably high rate. In contrast, many vaccination programmes have been highly successful and with our increase in knowledge of how vaccines work it will become increasingly feasible to develop design strategies for new vaccines based on a firm understanding of the molecular structures and cellular processes involved.

Vaccinology is not the province of any single discipline and requires contributions from chemistry, physics, biochemistry, genetics, immunology and epidemiology as well as virology, bacteriology and parasitology. The authors hope that this book will stimulate young scientists from all disciplines to consider the potential of vaccines in human and veterinary medicine for the next century and provoke thoughtful discussion on how best to exploit our increasing knowledge of pathogenic agents and the immune system in our continuing struggle against infectious diseases.

SUGGESTED READING

Brown F (1990) Modern approaches to vaccine. In: *Seminars in Virology*, Vol. 1, No. 1, 1990. Philadelphia: Saunders.

Almond JW and Burke KL (1990) Poliovirus as a vector for the presentation of foreign antigens. In: *Seminars in Virology*, Vol. 1, No. 1, pp. 11–20.

Mackett M, Smith GL and Moss B (1982) Vaccinia virus: a selectable eukaryotic cloning and expression vector. *Pro. Natl Acad. Sci. USA*, **79**, 7415–7419.

Mackett M (1990) Vaccinia virus as a vector for delivering foreign antigens. In: *Seminars in Virology*, Vol. 1, No. 1, pp. 39–48.

Morein B, Fossum C, Lovgren K and Hoglund S (1990) The iscom: a modern approach to vaccines. In: *Seminars in Virology*, Vol. 1, No. 1, pp. 49–56.

Panicali D and Paoletti E (1982) Construction of poxviruses as cloning vectors: insertion of the thymidine kinase gene from herpes virus into DNA of infectious vaccinia virus. *Pro. Natl Acad. Sci. USA*, **79**, 4927–4931.

Racaniello VR and Baltimore D (1981) Cloned poliovirus complementary DNA is infectious in mammalian cells. *Science* **214**, 916–919.

Glossary

α-Helix

Rod-like protein structure in which the inner core is formed by the tightly coiled α-carbon chain and the side chains protrude outwards in a helical way.

Amphipathicity

The property that hydrophobic residues cluster on one side of an α-helix and hydrophilic residues on the opposite side.

Antigen-presenting cell (APC)

A cell type, e.g. macrophage or dendritic cell, that is capable of presenting peptide antigens in association with major histocompatibility antigen to T-cells in a form recognisable by lymphocytes.

Antigenic drift

Process whereby by missense mutations in antigenic proteins of an organism slowly make it less able to be recognised by the immune system of the host.

Antigenic index

A composite measure of antigenicity of a particular stretch of amino acids in the primary sequence of a protein calculated from the hydropathy, flexibility, surface probability and secondary structure predicted for that set of residues.

Antigenic shift

A process whereby major antigenic proteins of viruses (especially influenza viruses) are changed dramatically by reassortment of genome fragments to give new strains to which no immunity exists in the host.

Antigenic site

A part of a protein to which one or more antibodies can bind, i.e. a number of related epitopes.

Attenuation

See live-attenuated vaccine.

Baculoviruses

Viruses that infect insects and are surrounded in the cells by a large amount of a polyhedral protein. This provides an excellent expression system.

β-Microglobulin

A 12 Kd protein found in the serum as well as in association with the major histocompatibility Class I antigens.

β-Sheet

A 'flat' protein protein structure in which the α carbon chain is almost fully extended and in which the side groups from one chain in the sheet interact with those of another (parallel or antiparallel) through hydrogen bonds.

Cercaria

Larval stage of a trematode which will develop into an adult.

Chimaeric viruses

A name commonly used in reference to hybrid agents produced by genetic engineering.

Chromium release assay

Assay for cell killing by T lymphocytes involving the loading of the target (antigen bearing cells) with radio-active chromium which is released when the target cell is killed (the process is MHC restricted).

Clones (bacterial)

A population of cells each derived from a single parental cell and having an identical genetic make-up. In recombinant DNA methodology often refers to cells which carry identical recombinant molecules.

Conformational epitope

An epitope that is formed by bringing together amino acid residues through folding of the α-carbon chain of a protein or through interaction of protein molecules in homo- or hetero-oligomers.

Cos sites

The single-stranded overhangs at the ends of λ DNA. They are capable of base pairing together to circularise the genome.

Cosmid vectors

Plasmid vectors into which the cos sites from λ bacteriophage have been inserted. Foreign DNA of up to 40 KB can be inserted and the resulting recombinant DNA can be in vitro packaged similar to λ bacteriophage DNA.

Cytokine

A soluble protein molecule which can alter the activity of cells.

Dead vaccine

A vaccine preparation which contains either the inactivated infectious agent or subunits of it (cf. Live-attenuated vaccine).

ELISA

Enzyme Linked Immunosorbent Assay; a test in which the amount of a protein bound to a solid support, usually consisting of microtitre plates, is assayed through its ability to bind another protein or antibodies the amounts of which can then be assayed by binding of a (second) antibody to which an enzyme is covalently linked. The amount of enzyme is assayed through conversion of a chromogenic substrate.

Endemic immunity

The acquisition of an immune status by natural means without the intervention of direct vaccination.

Enterotoxigenic

Producing a toxic effect in the gastrointestinal tract

Epitope

The part of an antigen that binds directly to the paratope of an antibody or T cell receptor.

Fimbrial

Proteinaceous structures external to the cell wall of bacteria.

Flexibility

A measure of the temperature factors, i.e. the amount by which the position of atoms in a given amino acid residue changes as a function of the temperature of a protein crystal.

Haemagglutinin

The protein with the ability of viruses and bacteria to agglutinate red blood cells.

Hepatosplenomegaly

Enlargement of the spleen and liver.

Histocompatibility antigens

Proteins involved in the self/non-self recognition to ensure that immune attacks are directed against foreign invaders and not against own tissues. There are two types of molecules class I and II interacting with different types of lymphocytes. These are referred to as the major histocompatibility complex (MHC).

Hydropathy	See Hydrophobicity.
Hydrophilicity	Love of water, the extent to which amino acid residues are likely to be in contact with water molecules.
Hydrophobicity	Also hydropathy: fear of water, the extent to which amino acid residues are likely to be on the inside of protein molecules, not exposed to water molecules.
Hypergammaglobulinaemia	Elevated levels of immunoglobulins seen in the serum.
λ Insertion vectors	λ bacteriophage vectors with unique restriction sites in the central part which allow insertion of up to 7–8 kb of foreign DNA.
λ Replacement vectors	λ bacteriophage vectors from which a central non-essential 'stuffer region' can be removed allowing the insertion of up to 20 kb of foreign DNA.
Langerhans cell	Antigen-presenting cell found in the skin.
Linear epitope	An epitope consisting of a small number of consecutive amino residues in the primary sequence of a protein.
Live-attenuated vaccine	A strain of virus (or bacterium) which usually by passage in other than the normal host or tissue culture cells or eggs has lost its virulence for the original host.
Merozoite	Stage in the development of protozoan parasites; in malaria released from liver cells (hepatocytes).
Monoclonal antibodies	Identical antibody molecules produced by the progeny of a (cloned) single cell resulting from the fusion of a myeloma cell line with spleen cells from an immunised animal (generally mouse).
Monoclonal antibody escape mutants	Mutant viruses with a changed amino acid at an epitope recognised by a monoclonal

antibody in the parental virus thus allowing the escape from neutralisation by that antibody.

Mycoplasma

Genus of bacteria lacking a cell wall, grown in association with eukaryotic cells.

Mucosal immune system

Lymphoid tissue associated with the mucosal surfaces of gastrointestinal tract, bronchus and genital tracts.

Neuraminidase

The protein with the enzymatic activity to cleave sialic acid residues from carbohydrate side chains often attached to glycoproteins.

Oncosphere

Infective stage of cestode parasites. It penetrates the host's small intestine and migrates to the tissue location in which the mature infective larva will develop.

Paratope

The antigen combining site of an antibody.

Parenteral vaccination

Vaccination through administration by a means other than absorption from the gastro-intestinal tract.

Phagemid

A plasmid vector housing the origin of replication of a single-stranded DNA bacteriophage. Infection of *E. coli* cells with helper phage allows the production of single-stranded DNA from the vector which can be used for sequencing or site-directed mutagenesis experiments.

Picornaviruses

Members of a family of small positive stranded RNA viruses some of which cause disease. The better known members of the group include the polioviruses, the common cold viruses (rhinoviruses) and the foot-and-mouth disease viruses.

Plasmid vectors

Double-stranded circular DNA molecules which replicate independently of the *E. coli* chromosome. They bear a marker for cells containing them, are generally present in high copy number and can house up to 10 kb of foreign DNA.

Polymerase chain reaction   A means of amplifying a specific DNA seg-
 (PCR)   ment from a large amount (e.g. human geno-
                               mic DNA) of DNA. Primers complementary
                               to flanking regions of the required sequence
                               are used. Following denaturation of the DNA
                               at high temperatures and annealing of the
                               primers, primer extension is carried out using
                               heat stable polymerases. Repeated rounds of
                               denaturation, annealing and primer extension
                               produce exponential amounts of product.

Sporozoite   Infective stage of protozoan parasites, in
                               malaria is inoculated along with mosquito
                               saliva and infects hepatocytes.

Stuffer fragment   The central non-essential region of some λ
                               bacteriophage vectors which can be excised
                               from λ replacement vectors allowing the
                               insertion of up to 20 kb of foreign DNA.

Thymus   Primary lymphoid organ in which T lympho-
                               cytes (T-cells) mature to functional subsets.

Western blot   A sideways transfer of proteins separated
                               by gel electrophoresis onto a solid support
                               so that their presence can be assessed by
                               immunological or specific staining reactions
                               or by interactions with other macromolecules
                               that contain reporter groups.

Index

Index compiled by Liza Weinkove